D0391690

THE HEALING POWER OF ILLNESS

German born **Thorwald Dethlefsen** is probably best known as a spiritual psychologist. He combines the qualifications of a trained psychologist with the insight gained through a deep study of the spiritual traditions. He runs a private institute in Munich as well as holding regular courses and speaking at lectures and conferences worldwide. Along with his co-author Rüdiger Dahlke MD, his work opens up completely new areas of thought regarding the understanding of illness.

By the same author
The Challenge of Fate

The Healing Power of Illness

*The Meaning of Symptoms and
How to Interpret Them*

Thorwald Dethlefsen

Rüdiger Dahlke MD

Translated by Peter Lemesurier

ELEMENT

Shaftesbury, Dorset ● Rockport, Massachusetts
Brisbane, Queensland

© C. Bertelsmann Verlag GmbH, München 1983
English translation © Peter Lemesurier 1990

This edition first published in 1990 by
Element Books Limited
Shaftesbury, Dorset

First published in the USA in 1991 by
Element, Inc.
42 Broadway, Rockport, MA 01966

First published in Australia in 1993 by
Element Books Limited for
Jacaranda Wiley Limited
33 Park Road, Milton, Brisbane 4064

Reprinted 1991
Reprinted 1992
Reprinted 1993
Reprinted January and October 1994

All rights reserved.
No part of this book may be
reproduced or utilized in any form or by any means,
electronic or mechanical, without permission
in writing from the Publisher.

Designed by Jenny Liddle
Cover design by Max Fairbrother
Cover illustration by Georgia O'Keefe, *Blue and Green Music*. 1919,
oil on canvas, 23 X 19", © 1990 The Art Institute of Chicago. All rights reserved.
Typeset by Footnote Graphics, Warminster, Wiltshire
Printed and bound in Great Britain by
Redwood Books, Trowbridge, Wiltshire

British Library Cataloguing in Publication Data
Dethlefsen, Thorwald
The healing power of illness.
1. Medicine, Psychosomatic
I. Title II. Dahlke, Rudiger
616.08

Library of Congress data available

ISBN 1–85230–123–6

Table of Contents

Contents

Foreword

This is an uncomfortable book, in that it deprives people of illness as an alibi for their unresolved problems. We propose to show that the patient is not the innocent victim of some quirk of nature, but actually the author of his or her own sickness. Thus, we shall not be addressing ourselves to environmental pollution, the ills of civilisation, unhealthy living or similar familiar scapegoats; instead we propose to bring the metaphysical aspect of illness to the fore. From this viewpoint symptoms are seen to be bodily expressions of psychological conflicts, able through their symbolism to reveal the patient's current problems.

In the first part of this book we therefore present the theoretical presuppositions underlying this approach and expound a philosophy of illness.

We recommend strongly that this first part be read carefully and in detail – possibly more than once – before turning to Part 2. This book could be described as a continuation or even elaboration of the previous book *The Challenge of Fate* (Coventure, 1984), although we have taken pains to give this new book its own self-contained identity. Nevertheless we would recommend *The Challenge of Fate* as good preparatory or even complementary reading, especially should the theoretical part of the present book pose any difficulties.

In Part 2 the most common disease-symptoms are presented in their symbolic aspects and interpreted as expressions of psychological problems. An index of individual symptoms at the end of the book will enable the reader to refer back to any given symptom as the need arises. Nevertheless it is our primary aim to use our explanations as a means of teaching readers a new way of seeing which will enable them to recognise the meanings of symptoms and develop their own interpretations for themselves. At the same time we have used the subject of illness as a hat-peg for a whole range of philosophical and esoteric themes whose application goes far beyond the narrow remit of mere illness.

This is not a difficult book, but at the same time it is not as simple or banal as it may seem to those who do not understand our basic concept. This book is not 'scientific', in that it lacks the caution necessarily involved in any 'scientific presentation'. It has been written for people who are prepared to set out on a path, and not merely to sit on the fence and waste time juggling with empty phrases. People whose goal is enlightenment have no time for rationalist science: what they need is knowledge. This book will run into a good deal of opposition, and yet at the same time we hope that it will reach those (be they few or many) who actually want to use it as an aid along their way. They, and only they, are the people for whom it is written.

The Authors
Munich, February 1983

Part One

Theoretical Preconditions for Understanding Sickness and Healing

One

Illness and Symptoms

Human understanding
Cannot grasp true instruction.
But if you are in doubt
And do not understand
You may happily discuss things
With me.

Yoka Daishi: 'Shodoka'

We are living at a time when modern medicine constantly presents the marvelling layman with fresh evidence of its almost miraculous skills and powers. At the same time, though, those who have a basic mistrust of modern medicine and its near omnipotence are raising their voices ever more loudly. An ever-growing number of people place a good deal more confidence in natural healing methods (be they very ancient or quite modern) or in homoeopathic therapies than in today's highly scientific orthodox medicine, which offers a whole range of targets for criticism – side-effects, symptom-shifts, lack of humanity, rocketing costs and much else besides. Yet what is a good deal more interesting than the details of the criticism is the fact that it occurs at all. For even before a criticism can be reduced to rational form it emerges as a vague feeling that something is no longer as it should be, and that the chosen way, despite – or even directly because of – its thorough-going application, is not leading to the hoped-for goal. This uneasiness about medical practice is an experience common to large numbers of people, including many younger doctors. Yet the concensus quickly disappears as soon as it comes to proposing new, alternative solutions. Some see salvation in the socialisation of medicine, others in replacing chemotherapy with natural and plant-based remedies. While some see research into earthly radiations as the key to solving all the problems, others swear by homoeopathy. Acupuncturists and reflexologists do their best to turn our medical gaze from mere morphological phenomena towards a more energy-orientated view of the overall body process. Perhaps the best way of summing up all the alternative methods and initiatives is to speak of a 'holistic' form of medicine – thus bearing witness to the endeavour not only to remain open to all the various approaches, but above all not to lose sight of the *whole* person as a psychosomatic unity. The fact that academic medicine *has* lost sight of it has in the meantime become obvious to nearly everybody. Its high specialisation and reliance on analysis as the basic principle of its research has inevitably resulted not only in an ever-greater and more exact knowledge of detail but also, at one and the same time, in its losing sight of the picture as a whole.

If we consider the immensely refreshing discussion and movement that is currently going on within medicine, it soon becomes clear that the talk is largely confined to the various methods and their effects, while little is so far being said about the theory or philosophy of medicine itself. Admittedly medicine lives in large measure by concrete, practical procedures, yet every procedure is – consciously or unconsciously – an expression of the philosophy on which it is based. The rock on which the ship of modern medicine is foundering is in no sense the efficacy of its procedures, but the view of life on which it has based those procedures, often without either discussion or reflection. It is in philosophy that it is failing – or rather lacking. Medical procedures have been founded up to now upon considerations of practicality and effectiveness, but medicine's inner 'lack of soul' has in the end brought down upon itself the accusation of inhumanity. True, this inhumanity expresses itself in many concrete, exterior forms, but the problem is not to be resolved by further changes of procedure. Many symptoms bear witness to the fact that medicine, too, is sick. The 'patient' that is medicine itself cannot be cured by tinkering around with the symptoms, any more than can any other patient. Notwithstanding this, most of those who criticise academic medicine and who champion alternative therapies take on board as a matter of course the philosophy and goals of academic medicine, and so apply their energies purely to changing its forms and methods.

It is the aim of this book to get to grips all over again with the problem of illness and healing. In no way, though, shall we be taking on board the familiar, received basic values that are universally held in this field to be so irrefutable. To be sure, this attitude will make our enterprise difficult and dangerous, for we cannot help but probe deeply and mercilessly into areas which are taboo even to the public at large. We are fully aware that we are undertaking a step which is certainly not the next one on medicine's planned developmental agenda. Indeed, it would be more accurate to say that there are a whole range of steps which have yet to be undertaken by established medical practice, yet whose deep understanding is a vital precondition for realising the concept that is basic to this book. Therefore we shall be addressing our presentation not so much towards the development of medicine in general, as to individual people whose powers of personal insight place them somewhat in advance of the rather sluggish general trend.

What goes on at the practical level never has any meaning in itself. The meaning of an event only emerges as a result of interpreting it, since it is the interpretation which alone enables us to experience it as *meaning-ful*. Thus, for example, the rising of a mercury column in a glass tube is, by itself, absolutely meaningless: only when we have interpreted the event as the expression of a change in temperature does the process become meaningful. The moment people cease to interpret world events and the outworkings of their own personal destiny, their existence sinks into meaninglessness and senselessness. But in order to interpret anything, we need a frame of reference which lies beyond the level at which whatever we are trying to interpret is manifesting itself. Consequently the events and initiatives of the material world – the world of forms – can be interpreted only by bringing in some metaphysical reference-system. Only when the visible world of forms 'becomes like an allegory', as Goethe puts it, does it acquire sense and meaning for people. Just as letters and numbers are formal vehicles for the ideas which underlie them, so everything *visible*, everything concrete and functional, is purely an expression of an idea, and thus a mediator of the invisible. In short, we can equally well refer to these two spheres as 'form' and 'content'. It is through form that content expresses itself, and it is in this way that forms become *meaning-ful*. Written signs or letters that convey no ideas and no meaning remain for us senseless and void. Even the most detailed analysis of them cannot alter the fact. The relationship between form and content is just as universally clear and understandable in the artistic context. The quality of a painting does not reside in the quality of the canvas or paints: the material components of the painting are merely vehicles and mediators of an idea which is the artist's inner picture. The function of the canvas and paints is thus to make it possible for the otherwise invisible to become visible, and so they are physical expressions of a metaphysical content.

These simple examples represent our attempt to bridge any gap in understanding which may surround the method applied in this book, a move to consider the themes of illness and healing in a *meaning-ful* way. But in the process we are quite deliberately and unequivocally leaving the sphere of 'scientific medicine' behind. We make no claim to be 'scientific' for the simple reason that our point of departure is a quite different one – a fact which means that scientific discussion or criticism of our approach is bound to miss the mark. Consequently it is with all due deliberation that we shall be abandoning the scientific framework, since this confines itself specifically to the functional level and thus makes it impossible for sense or meaning to become clear. Such an approach is not designed for inveterate rationalists and materialists: it *is* designed, though, for people who are ready to follow the intricate and by no means always logical paths of human consciousness. Among the most helpful companions on such a journey through the human soul are pictorial thinking, fantasy, association, irony and an ear for the linguistic background. And our chosen way demands not least the ability to tolerate paradox and ambivalence without immediately feeling obliged to destroy one pole or the other for the sake of imposing clarity.

In medicine, as in common speech, people refer to a whole variety of '*illnesses*'. This is an example of linguistic slovenliness which reveals very clearly the widespread misunderstanding which surrounds the concept of illness. 'Illness' is a term which can in fact only be used in the singular. The plural, 'illnesses', is just as meaningless as the plural of 'health' – 'healths'. Illness and health are singular concepts, since they refer to a human state or condition and not, as is fashionable in today's usage, to organs or parts of the body. The body is never ill or healthy, for it does no more than express messages from our consciousness. The body does nothing of itself, as anybody can confirm for himself by looking at a corpse. For its operation the body of a living person has two immaterial entities to thank – precisely those to which we generally refer as consciousness (soul) and life (spirit). It is consciousness which presents us with the messages that are manifested in the body and so eventually made visible. Consciousness is to the body as a radio programme is to the receiver. Since consciousness represents a non-material, self-sufficient quality in its own right, it is naturally neither a product of the body nor dependent on its existence.

Everything that happens within the body of a living being is the expression of a corresponding information pattern, or a condensation of a corresponding image (the Greek for 'image' is *eidolon*, which is also related to the concept 'idea'). When pulse and heart are following a particular rhythm, when the body temperature is being maintained at a constant level, when the glands are pumping out hormones, or when antibodies are being formed, these functions cannot be explained purely in material terms. Instead, each is dependent on a corresponding information pattern whose source is consciousness itself. When the multifarious bodily functions are chiming together in a particular way an overall pattern emerges which we feel to be harmonious and so refer to as *health*. If a particular function goes wrong, it compromises the overall harmony to a greater or lesser extent, and we call the result *illness*.

Illness, then, means the abandonment of harmony or the throwing into question of a hitherto balanced regime (we shall be seeing later that – seen from another angle – illness, too, is actually the creation of a kind of balance). But the disturbance of this harmony takes place within consciousness, at the informational level, and merely manifests itself in the body. In this way the body is the representational or realisational aspect of consciousness, as well as of all the processes and changes that go on within consciousness. Thus, just as the entire material world is merely the stage on which the play of the archetypes takes on form and so becomes 'like a metaphor', so by the same token the material body is the stage on which the images of consciousness force their way into expression. Hence, if a person's consciousness falls into imbalance, the fact becomes visible and tangible in the form of bodily symptoms. That is why it is misleading to say that the body is ever ill – only people can be ill – even though the illness does show up in symptomatic form *within* the body. (When a tragedy is performed, after all, it is not the stage, but the play that is tragic!)

Symptoms are many and various, yet they are all expressions of one and the same event which we call 'illness', and which always occurs within a person's consciousness. Just as the body cannot live without consciousness, so it cannot become 'ill' without consciousness either.

At this point, meanwhile, it should be understood that we do not accept the nowadays customary division between somatic, psychosomatic and mental conditions. Such a concept is more likely to hinder the understanding of illness than to help it. True, our viewpoint does correspond somewhat to the psychosomatic model, yet with the difference that we take such a view of *all* symptoms without exception. The distinction between

7

'somatic' (i.e. bodily) and 'psychic' (i.e. psychological) can at best be applied to the level at which a symptom appears – but cannot be used to locate illness itself. The age-old concept of mental illness is completely misleading, since the mind (that is, the consciousness) can never become ill. Rather is it a case here of symptoms which manifest themselves on the psychological level – that is, which show up within a person's consciousness.

Consequently we shall be endeavouring here to develop a unitary view of illness which uses the distinction between 'somatic' and 'psychological' at most to refer to the primary level on which a symptom appears.

Given the conceptual distinction between illness (consciousness-level) and symptom (body-level), the focus of our consideration of illness will necessarily shift away from the familiar analysis of what is going on in the body to something which has hitherto been far from familiar, at least in this context – namely a thorough-going look at the psychological level. Thus, we shall be acting rather like a critic who, instead of panning a bad play in analytical terms or proposing changes of scenery, props or actors, turns his attention directly to the play itself.

When a symptom manifests itself in a person's body, it draws attention to itself to a greater or lesser degree and thus interrupts, often quite abruptly, life's former continuity. A symptom is a signal which directs our awareness, interest and energy to itself and in the process upsets the usual smooth flow of things. Willy nilly, a symptom demands our attention. We regard this interruption from 'out there' as a disturbance and therefore we generally have only one aim – to make what is troubling us (the 'trouble') go away again. People hate to be disturbed – and so the battle against the symptom begins. Even a battle, meanwhile, implies concern and attention – and so it is that the symptom always manages to ensure that we concern ourselves with it.

Ever since the time of Hippocrates, academic medicine has been trying to convince patients that a symptom is a more or less accidental phenomenon whose cause is to be sought in mechanical processes, and so everybody is eager to research those processes. Academic medicine carefully avoids *interpreting* the symptom, and so condemns both symptom and illness to meaninglessness. Yet this deprives the signal of its true function – for in the absence of symptoms the signals lose all significance.

By way of clarification, let us take an analogy. On its instrument panel a car has a whole range of warning-lights, which come on only when one of the car's vital functions is no longer operating properly. Yet in the actual event of one of them lighting up during a journey, we are far from happy about it. We feel obliged by this signal to interrupt our trip. In spite of our understandable disquiet, however, it would be stupid to get annoyed at the light itself. It is, after all, telling us about some happening which we otherwise would have taken much longer to find out about, since it lies in what for us is an 'invisible' zone. Consequently, we treat the fact that the light has come on as the cue to call a mechanic, with the object of ensuring that after he has done his job the light will no longer be on and we can happily resume our journey. Nevertheless, we should be pretty indignant if the mechanic were to achieve this end simply by taking out the light-bulb. True, the light would no longer be on – which would indeed be what we had wanted – but the way in which this had been achieved would appear to us to be far too superficial. Rather than stop the light coming on at all, we would regard it as far more sensible to make it unnecessary for it to light up in the first place. But for this to happen, we should need to shift our attention from the light itself and turn to what lies behind it, so as to find out what is actually out of order. The light's real function, in other words, is and was simply to act as an indicator and make us ask questions.

As is the warning-light to our example, so is the symptom to our subject. That which constantly reveals itself as a series of bodily symptoms is the visible expression of an invisible process; it is designed as a signal whose function is to stop us in our tracks, reveal that something is no longer in order and make us ask questions about what lies behind it all. Here, once again, it is silly to get upset about the symptom, and downright absurd to try to switch it off simply by preventing it from appearing. The symptom has to be made superfluous, not prevented. But in order to do this it is just as necessary as before for us to avert our gaze from the symptom itself and examine things more deeply, if we are to understand what the symptom is really pointing to.

It is in its incompetence to undertake this step, however, that the main problem of academic medicine lies: it is far too mesmerised by the symptoms themselves. Consequently it equates symptom with illness – in other words it is unable to distinguish form from content. It then goes on to apply enormous resources and skills to the treatment of organs and parts of the body – but never of the actual person who is ill. It chases after the goal of one day being able to do away with symptoms altogether, without for a moment looking more deeply into the sense or feasibility of the idea. It is astonishing how impotent even plain facts are to bring this euphoric wild-goose-chase back down to earth. Since the advent of so-called modern, scientific medicine the number of patients has not gone down even by the smallest fraction of one per cent. True, efforts are made to mask this sobering fact with the aid of statistics that refer only to particular groups of symptoms. Thus, victory is proudly proclaimed over the infectious diseases, for example, without a word about what other symptoms have increased in intensity and frequency over the same period.

No honest view can emerge until people start to look not at the symptoms, but at illness as such – and this has not declined, and will assuredly not decline in the future. Illness is as deeply rooted in human nature as death itself, and is not to be eradicated from the world by a few mere mechanical gimmicks. Were we to appreciate illness and death in all their awesome greatness, we should realise in the light of that appreciation how laughable our ill-begotten efforts are to pit our powers against them. But then, of course, we can always shield ourselves from any such disillusionment by explaining away illness and death as mere physical processes, so making it possible at the same time still to believe in our own greatness and authority.

To sum up thus far, then: illness is a human condition which indicates that the patient is no longer *in order* or *in harmony* at the level of consciousness. This loss of inner balance manifests itself in the body as a symptom. The symptom is at one and the same time a signal and a vehicle of information, for its appearance interrupts our life's familiar flow and forces us to give the symptom our attention. The symptom alerts us to the fact that we are sick people or sick souls – that is, we have lost our inner, psychological balance. The symptom tells us so: it says that something is missing. 'What's a*miss*?', people used at one time to ask those who were ill – though the latter always replied by saying what they *had*: 'I've got a pain.'* Nowadays we have taken to asking straight out, 'What have you got?' On closer consideration, the mutual polarity of these two questions – 'What's amiss?' and 'What have you got?' – is very revealing. Both are entirely appropriate from the patient's point of view. Anybody who is ill is lacking something, and specifically at the consciousness level: if they were not lacking something they would be whole – both healthy and complete. On the other hand, once that wholeness is compromised in some respect,

To this day sufferers in Scotland are routinely asked, 'What are you lacking?' – tr.

then they are 'un-whole' – that is, unwell or ill. This 'ill-ness' shows up in the body as a symptom, which is something that one *has*. And so it comes about that what one *has* is an expression of what one *lacks*. One lacks some aspect of consciousness, and therefore has a symptom.

Once people have grasped the difference between illness and symptom, their basic attitude and approach to illness becomes transformed at a stroke. No longer do they see the symptom as the great enemy which it is their highest goal to resist and destroy. Instead they discover in the symptom a partner capable of helping them to discover what they lack and so to overcome their current illness. At this point the symptom becomes a kind of teacher, helping us take responsibility for our own development and the growth of our consciousness – a teacher, though, who can show great severity and harshness should we fail to respect what is in fact our highest law. Illness knows only one goal: to make us become whole.

In the course of this quest the symptom can tell us what we are lacking thus far. This presupposes, however, that we understand the language of symptoms. It is the re-learning of this language of symptoms that is the purpose of this book – re-learning, because this language has existed from the earliest times, and is therefore not to be discovered, but *re*-discovered. Our whole language is psychosomatic – which is to say that it knows all about the connections between body and psyche. If we can learn once again to appreciate our language's capacity for *double entendre*, to listen in to its ulterior meanings, then we shall very soon be able to hear what our symptoms have to say and learn to understand them. Our symptoms have more – and more important – things to say to us even than our fellow human beings do, for they are far more intimate associates, pertain to us alone and are unique in really knowing us from the inside.

The result, however, is a degree of honesty that is not all that easy to put up with. Even our best friends would never dare tell us the truth about ourselves to our face in the honest, unvarnished way that our symptoms always do. No wonder, then, that we have allowed ourselves to forget the language of symptoms: it is, after all, always easier to be dishonest. Yet merely refusing to listen or understand will not make the symptoms go away. We are constantly forced to come to terms with them in one way or another. If only we can dare to listen to them and enter into communication with them, they will become incorruptible teachers and guides along our way towards true healing. By telling us what we are currently lacking, by making us aware of whatever themes we still have to integrate consciously within ourselves, they give us the opportunity, through a process of learning and inner awakening, to render the symptoms superfluous.

It is here that the difference lies between *fighting* illness and *transmuting* illness. Healing arises exclusively from the transmutation of illness, never from conquering symptoms. For, as the linguistic wisdom reveals, healing presupposes that the patient has become 'healthier' – which is to say 'more whole' or 'more complete' (our use of the 'ungrammatical' comparative form of *whole* simply implies *nearer to wholeness*: the comparative is actually no more legitimate where health is concerned, either!) Healing always means a closer approach to the whole – to that wholeness of consciousness which is also known as enlightenment. Healing occurs through the incorporation of that which is missing, and thus is not possible without an expansion of consciousness. Illness and healing are twin concepts which have relevance only to consciousness and are not applicable to the body, since a body itself can be neither ill nor healthy. All that it can do is reflect the corresponding states and conditions of consciousness itself.

But it is precisely over this point that academic medicine is most liable to criticism. It talks of 'healing' without paying due heed to the one level on which healing is actually possible. True, it is not our intention here to criticise how medicine goes about its job when it is making no specific claim to healing as such. Medical practice confines itself to purely practical measures which in themselves are neither 'good' nor 'bad' but are simply available forms of intervention on the material level. On this level medicine is often extraordinarily effective, and so turning its methodology into a kind of general bogeyman is something which is best reserved for oneself, not imposed on other people. It all depends, after all, on just how prone one is to try and change the world by brute force, or on whether one has managed to unmask such an approach – for oneself, at least – as the illusion it is. Those who have seen through the game have absolutely no obligation to go on playing it (even though there is absolutely nothing to stop them either!), but nevertheless they have no right to deny it to others merely because they themselves no longer need it. Even learning to cope with an illusion can in the event have its benefits too.

Thus, we are less concerned here with what people do, than with their *awareness* of what they do. Readers who have understood our viewpoint thus far will note at this point that our criticism naturally applies just as much to 'natural' healing methods as to academic medicine itself. Natural methods, after all, likewise attempt to bring about 'healing' and to prevent illness through practical intervention, as well as talking about a 'healthy lifestyle'. The underlying philosophy is thus identical to that of academic medicine, but for the fact that the methods involved are somewhat less noxious and more natural. (Homoeopathy, which belongs strictly neither to academic medicine nor to naturopathy, may be seen as an exception to this.)

Humanity's path is one that leads from the unhealthy to the healthy, from illness to that true healing which is also whole-ness and even *holi*-ness. Illness is not some accidental, and therefore disagreeable upset along the way, but the very way itself along which people can progress towards wholeness. The more consciously we can think about that way, the more likely is it to lead us to the goal. Our purpose is not to resist illness but to use it. Nevertheless, if we are to succeed in doing so, we are now going to need to go into things somewhat more deeply.

Two

Polarity and Unity

Jesus said to them: When you make the two
as one and when you make the inner as the outer
and the outer as the inner and the above
as the below and when you make the male and
the female as a single one, so that the male
is not male and the female not female,
when you make eyes in place of an eye
and a hand in place of a hand and a foot in
place of a foot, an image in place of an image,
then you will enter the kingdom.

Gospel of Thomas, Log.22

We now feel obliged once again to tackle a subject already broached in *The Challenge of Fate* – namely the problem of polarity. While on the one hand we are anxious to avoid tedious repetition, on the other hand an understanding of polarity is an essential precondition for pursuing our line of thought any further. In fact, in the last analysis, it would be difficult to over-concern ourselves with polarity, since it presents us with the central problem of our very existence.

The moment we say the word 'I', we immediately cut ourselves off from everything that we experience as 'Not-I', or 'you' – and with this step we become prisoners of polarity. Henceforth our 'I' shackles us to the world of opposites, which is divided not only into 'I' and 'you', but also into inner and outer, man and woman, good and bad, right and wrong, and so on. Our human ego makes it impossible for us to perceive, or even imagine, unity or wholeness in any form whatsoever. Our consciousness splits and dissects everything into pairs of opposites which, the moment we come face to face with them, we experience as conflicts. They force us to decide, and thus to come to a *de-cision*, a cutting-apart. Our intellect does nothing but constantly cut up reality into ever smaller pieces ('analysis') and then distinguish between the resultant bits (the 'power of discrimination'). We say yes to the one and no to its opposite – for 'opposites (as we say) are mutually exclusive'. Yet with every no, with every *ex-clusion*, we reinforce our *un-whole-ness*, for in order to be whole it is necessary for us to lack nothing. Perhaps it is already becoming evident, then, how intimately the subject of illness and healing is connected with the concept of polarity. Indeed, the idea can be formulated even more explicitly: illness is polarity, healing is the transcending of polarity.

Behind the polarity that we encounter as human beings there stands a unity – that all-embracing unity within which the opposites lie as yet undifferentiated from each other. This level of being is also referred to as the All – an All which by definition includes everything, with the result that there can be nothing outside this unity, this All. Within this unity there is neither alteration nor change nor development, for it is subject neither to time nor to space. The All-Oneness is in a state of eternal rest; it is pure Being, without form or activity. It should be evident, then, that anything we say about the Oneness has to be expressed in negative terms – that is, by negating something: 'without time', 'without space', 'without change', 'without end'.

Every positive statement is a product of our divided world and is for that reason not applicable to the Oneness. From the viewpoint of our polar consciousness the Oneness therefore appears as *No-thing*. This formulation is perfectly correct, yet it often causes us as human beings to jump to false conclusions. Westerners in particular generally feel let down and frustrated to learn, for example, that the meaning of *nirvana*, the state of consciousness which is the goal of Buddhist philosophy, is for all intents and purposes nothing (literally 'extinction'). The human ego always loves to feel that there is something that lies outside itself, and is most reluctant to understand that it must actually be extinguished if it is to become one with the All. In the Oneness Everything and No-thing are one. No-thing eschews all manifestation or definition and thus escapes polarity. This No-thing is the ultimate foundation of all being (the Ain Soph of the Kabbalists, the Tao of the Chinese, the Neti-Neti of the Hindus). It alone really exists, without beginning or end, from eternity to eternity.

We can refer to this Oneness, but we cannot imagine it. Unity is the polar opposite of polarity itself, and is therefore an idea that challenges our intellect – indeed, we can even sense and experience it to some degree through certain exercises or meditation-techniques that help us develop the ability to unify our consciousness, at least for short spells. Nevertheless it always eludes linguistic description or intellectual analysis, since our thought specifically demands polarity as a condition for its own operation. Without polarity, without the division into subject and object, into knower and known, knowledge itself is impossible. In the Oneness there is no knowledge, but only being. In the Oneness all desire, all wanting and striving, all movement ceases – for there is no more 'out there' to hanker after. It is the old paradox that only in no-thing is plenty to be found.

Let us then return to the sphere of existence which we certainly *can* experience. We all have a polar consciousness which contrives to ensure that the world appears to us in polar form. It is vital to get firmly into our minds that it is not the world, but the consciousness with which we view the world that is polar. As an example of the laws of polarity in action, let us consider the breath, which provides all of us with our basic experience of polarity. As the inbreath and outbreath constantly alternate, they create a rhythm. But rhythm is nothing more than a constant alternation between two poles. Rhythm is the basic pattern of all life. Physics suggests much the same, with its revelation that all phenomena can be reduced to vibrations. Destroy rhythm, and we destroy life, for life is rhythm. Anyone who refuses to breathe out can no longer breathe in. From this it is clear that the inbreath depends on the outbreath: it cannot exist without its polar opposite. The one pole depends for its life on the other. If we take one pole away, the other disappears also. In the same way, electricity arises from the tension between two poles – but if we take one pole away the electricity simply vanishes.

The illustration opposite is a long-familiar picture puzzle with the aid of which each of us can re-experience the problem for ourselves. In this case the polarity lies between foreground and background or, in more concrete terms, between 'faces' and 'vase'. Which particular figure I perceive out of the two possibilities depends on whether I take the white or the black area to be the background. If I interpret the dark area as background, then the white area becomes foreground, and I see a vase. But this perception is turned on its head if I make the white area the background, for then I see the black area as foreground, and what shows up is two faces in profile. This optical game gives us the chance to observe precisely what happens within us when we stand our perception on its head. The two pictorial elements of vase and faces are simultaneously inherent in the image as a single unity, yet force the observer to make and either/or

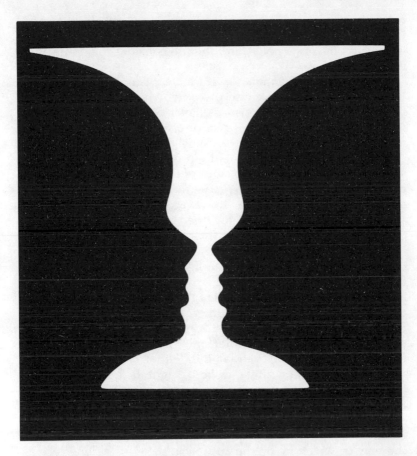

decision. Either we see the vase or we see the faces. It is easy enough to perceive both aspects of the image one after another, but it is very difficult simultaneously to hold both in our awareness with equal prominence.

This optical illusion offers us a good way-in to understanding polarity. In the picture the black pole is dependent on the white pole, and vice versa. Take one of the poles away (whether black or white makes no difference), and the whole image disappears *in both its aspects*. Here, once again, the black takes its life from the white, and the foreground from the background, just as does the inbreath from the outbreath or the positive electrical pole from the negative. This high degree of mutual dependence between two opposites shows us that behind every polarity there is an evident unity – though one which we humans, with our existing consciousness, are incapable of recognising or appreciating in all its oneness and simultaneity. Consequently we are forced to split every manifestation of the one reality into two poles, and then to consider them one after the other.

Indeed, this phenomenon is the very origin of time itself – that deceiver which likewise owes its existence exclusively to the polarity of our consciousness. Polarities burst forth from the womb of reality as twin aspects of one and the same unity – aspects, though, which we can only appreciate consecutively, one after the other. Consequently it depends on our particular standpoint which of the two sides of the coin we happen to see at any one time. Only by the superficial observer are polarities seen as mutually exclusive, however. Closer examination reveals that the polarities go together to make a unity and are dependent on one another for their very existence.

This fundamental realisation was first arrived at by science in the course of its research into light. At one time there were two opposing views about the nature of light rays: some advanced the wave-theory, others the particle-theory, and each theory seemed to exclude the other. If light consisted of waves, then it could not consist of particles, and vice versa: it was a case, in other words, of either/or. With the passage of time, however, it became clear that this 'either/or' was the wrong way of approaching the question. Light is both waves *and* particles. Indeed, let us stand the statement on its head: light is neither waves *nor* particles. Light, in its oneness, is ... light, and as such cannot be tied down by polar human consciousness at all. This light reveals itself to the observer only in relation to the way in which he or she approaches it – in the one case as waves, in the other as particles.

Polarity is like a door that has 'Entrance' written on one side of it and 'Exit' on the other: it remains one and the same door but, depending on which side we approach it from, we see only one of these twin aspects of it. It is out of this necessity of splitting unities into separate aspects and then considering them one at a time that time itself then arises, for it is only as a result of contemplating it with a polar consciousness that the *all-at-once-ness* of existence is transformed into a *one-thing-after-the-other-ness*. Just as unity stands behind polarity, so eternity stands behind time. But it should be borne in mind that the concept of eternity has the metaphysical sense of timelessness, and does not mean (as Christian theology has traditionally misunderstood it to mean) a long, unending continuum of time.

The way in which our consciousness and our drive to identify things splits primal unities into opposites is just as easy to observe when we look at ancient languages. People of earlier cultures seem to have been rather more successful at sensing the unity that underlies the polarities, for in ancient languages many words still have a basic bi-polarity. Only with the further development of language did these originally ambivalent words start to become assigned exclusively to one pole only, mainly with the aid of vowel-shifts and vowel-lengthenings. (Sigmund Freud himself was to recognise this phenomenon in his paper on the ambivalence of early vocabulary entitled *Gegensinn der Urworte*.)

Thus it is not difficult to recognise, for example, the common roots that link the Latin words *clamare* (to shout) and *clam* (softly), or *siccus* (dry) and *sucus* (juice); *altus*, in later no less than in earlier times, meant 'high' as well as 'deep'. In Greek, *pharmakon* meant 'poison' as well as 'medicine'. In German the words *stumm* (dumb) and *Stimme* (voice) are related, and in English this basic bi-polarity comes right out into the open in the word *without*, which contains within itself elements meaning both 'with' and 'without', even though nowadays the word as a whole is assigned to the one pole only. Even more germane to our theme is the linguistic relationship between the German words *bös* (bad) and *baß*. The word *baß* is Old High German and means something like 'good'. In modern German this word nowadays occurs only in the two combinations *fürbaß*, which means 'indeed', and *baß erstaunt*, which could be rendered as 'truly astonished'. The English word *bad* also derives from this same root, as well as the German words *Buße (penitence)* and *büßen* (to atone). This linguistic phenomenon, namely the original use of a single word to signify opposite poles – 'good' and 'bad', for example – shows graphically the way in which a common unity stands behind every polarity. The specific identification of good with bad is something into which we shall be looking very closely, and perhaps even at this stage it can make us aware of how immense the consequences are of understanding this whole subject of polarity.

We experience the polarity of our consciousness subjectively in the alternation of two clearly delineated states of consciousness, namely waking and sleeping. These two states of consciousness we are apt to see as inner analogues of the outer day/night polarity in nature. Thus, we quite frequently refer to our 'day-consciousness' and 'night-consciousness', or to the 'day' and 'night' sides of the soul. Closely associated with this polarity is the division between the conscious mind and the unconscious. Thus it is that during the daytime we think of that sphere of consciousness in which we spend our nights and out of which dreams arise as 'unconscious'. Strictly speaking, though, the word *un-conscious* is not a particularly appropriate term, since the prefix *un*–negates the word *conscious* which follows it – a negation which fails to fit the facts of the case. *Unconscious* is not the same as *consciousness-less*. It is just that in sleep we find ourselves in a different state of *conscious-ness*. There can, after all, be absolutely no question of a consciousness that is not there. The unconscious, then, is in no sense an absence of consciousness, but simply a piece of unilateral classification on the part of the daytime consciousness, which is aware that something seems to be there, but is unable to get a grasp of it. But why, in that case, do we identify ourselves so unquestioningly with the daytime consciousness?

Ever since the spread of depth psychology we have become accustomed to representing our consciousness in *stratified* form – distinguishing between a conscious, a subconscious and an unconscious mind. In fact, this way of organising the mind into 'upper' and 'lower' aspects is in no way a necessity of nature: it does, though, correspond to a symbolic way of relating to space which allocates sky and light to the 'upper' pole and earth and darkness to the 'lower' one. If we were to attempt a graphic model of such a view of human consciousness, we could present it in the following form:

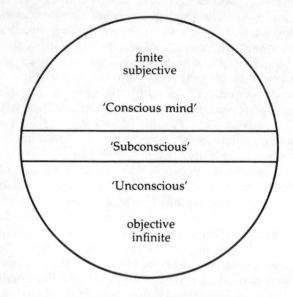

Here the circle symbolises consciousness itself which, being all-embracing, is non-finite and eternal. The circle's circumference should consequently not be seen as any kind of boundary, but simply as a symbol for the All-embracingness. From this, however, we are each cut off by our personal *I*, and thus arises a subjective, finite conscious mind. As a result of this we lose all access to the residual – that is, cosmic – consciousness. It is unknown to us: we are un-conscious of it. (C. G. Jung calls this level the 'collective unconscious'.) The dividing-line between the individual's *I* and the remaining 'sea of consciousness' is in no sense an absolute one, however: rather should it be seen as a kind of membrane which is permeable in both directions. This membrane corresponds to the subconscious. It bears within it not only contents that have sunk down into it from the conscious mind (i.e. been 'forgotten'), but also contents that are continually rising up out of the unconscious, such as premonitions, 'grand dreams', intuitions, visions and so on.

If we identify ourselves particularly strongly with our conscious mind alone, this very largely inhibits the permeability of the subconscious, for the unconscious contents are then perceived as being alien and therefore frightening. A greater degree of permeability can lead to a kind of 'mediumism'. But a state of enlightenment or 'cosmic consciousness' would only be attained by transcending the boundary altogether, so that conscious mind and unconscious become one. But then this step is synonymous with the annihilation of the *I*, whose very autonomy depends on the initial division. It is this step which, in Christian terminology, is described in the words: 'I (conscious mind) and my Father (unconscious) are one.'

Human consciousness finds its physical manifestation in the brain, within which the typically human power of discrimination and judgement is allocated to the cerebral cortex. No wonder, then, that the polarity of human consciousness finds its corresponding mark in the very anatomy of the cortex. It is a matter of common knowledge that the cortex is organised into two hemispheres, which are joined to each other by the so-called *corpus callosum*. In the past, medicine has attempted to treat various symptoms such as epilepsy or unbearable pain by surgically severing this organ and so cutting off all neural pathways between the two hemispheres ('commisurotomy').

Violent though such an intervention may appear, the operation seems at first sight to have no side-effects worth mentioning. This is how it was discovered that the two hemispheres apparently represent two totally self-sufficient brains, both capable of getting on with their job quite independently. However, once patients whose hemispheres had been separated in this way were subjected to more discriminating experimental conditions, it started to become ever more obvious that the two hemispheres differ very sharply from each other both in character and in jurisdiction. It is well-known, of course, that the neural pathways are 'cross-wired', with the result that the right side of the body is supplied with nerves from the left half of the brain and, conversely, the left half of the body from the right hemisphere. If the patients already described are now blindfolded and given, for example, a corkscrew to hold in the left hand, they are unable to *name* the object – that is, they cannot find the word that goes with the thing they are touching and feeling – yet have not the slightest difficulty in using it correctly. This situation is reversed if they are given the object to hold in their *right* hand: now they know the right name for it, but cannot figure out how to use it.

Just like the hands, the ears and eyes, too, are each connected to the opposite side of the brain. In another experiment, a variety of geometrical shapes were shown separately to the right and left eyes of a female patient whose *corpus callosum* had been severed. In the course of this, nude photographs were projected into the left eye's visual field in such a way as to be perceptible only to the right side of the brain. The patient blushed and giggled, but when asked by the leading experimenter what she had seen she replied, 'Nothing, just a flash of light,' and carried on giggling. Thus, an image perceived by the right hemisphere can produce a definite reaction, even though it is incapable of being perceived or defined in thought or word. Similarly, if smells are introduced only into the left nostril, a corresponding reaction takes place, even though the patient cannot identify the smell. If a compound word such as 'football' is shown to a patient in such a way that the left eye is given the first part – 'foot' – to look at, while the right is allocated only the second – 'ball', the patient reads only the word 'ball', since the word 'foot' cannot be analysed linguistically by the right half of the brain.

Such experiments have recently been elaborated and refined even further to the point where what has been established to date can be roughly summarised as follows: both halves of the brain are clearly differentiated from each other in their functions and capabilities, as well as in their respective areas of responsibility. The left hemisphere could be called the 'verbal' hemisphere, because it is responsible for logic and linguistic structure, for reading and for writing. It subdivides all our experience of the world analytically and rationally – that is, it thinks digitally. Consequently the left side of the brain is also responsible for counting and calculating. Moreover, our experience of time, too, has its seat in the left hemisphere.

At the same time all our bi-polar abilities are to be found in the *right* hemisphere: instead of analysis, what we find here is the ability instantly to grasp complex relationships, patterns and structures in their entirety. Thus, this half of the brain permits us to grasp the whole – the *Gestalt* – on the basis of a mere part (*pars pro toto*). It would seem that we also have the right half of the brain to thank for our ability to form and grasp those logical concepts which have no actual existence of their own – our higher concepts and abstractions. In the right brain, though, we find only the most archaic of speech-forms, which arrange themselves more on the basis of sound-patterns and associations than of syntax. Poetry and the speech of schizophrenics both give a good idea of the language of the right hemisphere. This is also where analogical thought and our handling of symbols are located. The right brain is responsible for the psyche's world of images and dreams and is not subject to the left hemisphere's sense of time.

Depending on what activity we are currently engaged in, one of the two hemispheres is always dominant. Thus, logical thought, reading, writing and calculating demand that the left hemisphere be in control, whereas when we are listening to music, dreaming, imagining or meditating it is the right hemisphere that is dominant. Despite the dominance at any given time of the one side of the brain, however, the healthy individual always has at his or her disposal the contents of the non-dominant side too, for a lively exchange of information is constantly passing across the *corpus callosum*. The polar specialisation of the twin hemispheres coincides with great exactness to the age-old esoteric teachings on polarity. In Taoism the two underlying principles into which the Oneness of the Tao divides itself were called yang (the masculine principle) and yin (the feminine principle). In the hermetic tradition the same polarity was expressed symbolically by sun (masculine) and moon (feminine). The Chinese yang, like the sun, in other words, is a symbol for the active, positive, masculine principle which corresponds in psychological terms to the daytime consciousness. The yin or lunar principle comprises the negative, feminine, receptive principle and corresponds to the individual's unconscious.

These classic polarities are not difficult to tie in with the actual results of scientific research. Thus, the left hemisphere is yang, masculine, active, conscious and corresponds to the sun-symbol – and thus to the individual's daytime aspect. And it is a fact that it is the left brain whose nerves are connected to the right side – the active or masculine side – of the body. The right hemisphere, by contrast, is yin, negative, feminine. It corresponds to the lunar principle – the individual's night-time aspect or

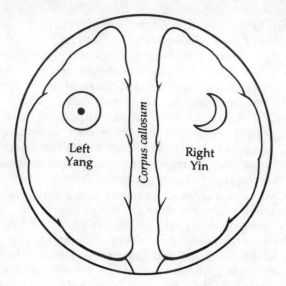

LEFT	RIGHT
Logic	Shape-recognition
Language (syntax, grammar)	All-in perception
	Spatial awareness
	Archaic speech-forms
Verbal hemisphere:	
Reading	Music
Writing	Smell
Calculating	Pattern
Counting	
Subdivision of environment	All-inclusive view of world
Digital thinking	Analogical thinking
Linear thought	Symbolism
Time-dependence	Timelessness
Analysis	Holism
	Logical concepts
Intelligence	Intuition

YANG	YIN
+	−
Sun	Moon
Masculine	Feminine
Day	Night
Conscious	Unconscious
Life	Death

LEFT	RIGHT
Activity	Passivity
Electric	Magnetic
Acid	Alkaline
Right side of body	Left side of body
Right hand	Left hand

unconscious – and accordingly is connected with the left-hand side of the body. For ease of reference the relevant terms and concepts are set out in tabular form above.

Certain modern schools of thought within psychology are already beginning to turn the old, horizontal, Freudian model of consciousness through ninety degrees, replacing the concepts 'conscious mind' and 'unconscious' with the left and right hemispheres respectively. This renaming, though, is purely a question of form and does little to alter content, as comparison with the diagrams overleaf will show. Both the horizontal and the vertical layouts are merely particular versions of the old Chinese symbol known as the *Tai Chi*, which subdivides the circle (signifying wholeness or unity) into a black and a white half, each of which contains in its turn a 'germ' of the opposite polarity in the form of a dot of the opposite colour. In a similar way, unity is divided by our consciousness into mutually complementary polarities.

It is not difficult to see how *unwhole* a person would be if he or she possessed only one of the two hemispheres; yet today's normal, scientific world-view is in reality just as unwhole, since it is that of the left side of the brain only. From this viewpoint everything has to be rational, reasonable and analytically tangible; only phenomena that are circumscribed by space and time

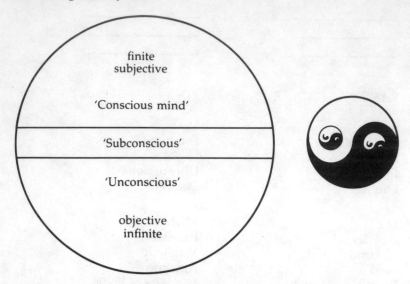

Horizontal model of consciousness

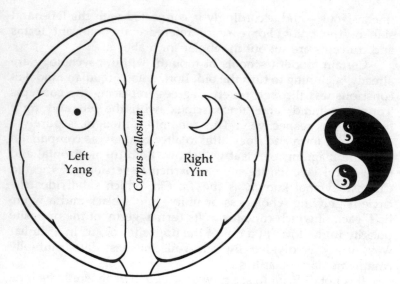

Vertical model of consciousness

can possibly exist. Yet such a view of the world is only half the truth, for it is the view of only half our consciousness – of only half the brain. All those contents of consciousness that people are so keen to dismiss as irrational, nonsensical, mystical, occult and fantastic are no more than opposite and complementary ways in which human beings are capable of viewing the world.

Just how different our assessments are of these two complementary viewpoints is evident from the fact that research into the abilities of the two halves of the brain was able very quickly to recognise and describe what the left brain does, while the fact that the right hemisphere seemed to have no logical function caused researchers to puzzle long and hard over its sense and purpose. Yet human nature itself places considerably more value on the skills of the right – or irrational – half of the brain: in life-threatening contexts it automatically switches over from left-brain dominance to right-brain dominance, since mere analytical procedures are not up to coping with such dangerous situations. With the right hemisphere in charge, we are given the chance to act calmly and competently thanks to its all-in mode of perception. It is to this switch-over, indeed, that the long-familiar phenomenon of the 'life-film' owes its existence. In the immediate proximity of death people are known to review their whole lives – to re-experience all the situations they have lived through once again – in a single flash. This phenomenon provides a good example of what we have already referred to as the 'timelessness' of the right brain.

In our view the real significance of brain-hemisphere theory lies in the fact that it could help science itself to realise how one-sided and partial its own view of the world has been up to now, and to learn through a study of the right brain how valid and necessary is that other way of viewing the world. At the same time it could learn from this very example that the law of polarity is the central law of all nature – for it is science's total inability to think analogically (that is, in right-brain mode) that has so far prevented any such step.

This same example, meanwhile, should clearly remind us once again of what the law of polarity involves: namely the splitting apart of unity by human consciousness into polar opposites. These two poles are mutually complementary (and compensatory), and each therefore needs the other as a condition for its existence. Polarity brings with it the inability to consider both aspects of a whole at the same time, and hence imposes on us that *one-thing-after-the-other-ness* which produces the phenomena of 'rhythm', 'time' and 'space'. Should a polar consciousness wish to reduce unity, or Oneness, to words, then it can do so only with the aid of paradox. The advantage that polarity bestows on us is the gift of *under-standing*, which is impossible without it. The aim and desire of a polar consciousness is to *over-come* its time-conditioned *un-whole-ness* and become healed – that is, whole – once more.

All paths of healing or initiation are but a single path that leads from polarity to unity. Yet the step from polarity to unity is such a radical, qualitative change that for a polar consciousness it is difficult if not impossible to imagine. Every metaphysical system, religion or esoteric school teaches exclusively this self-same path from duality to unity. From this it necessarily follows that all these teachings are concerned, not with 'improving the world', but with 'leaving the world behind'.

It is precisely this point that is the great target for the many critics and opponents of such teachings. Pointing to all the world's needs and injustices, they reproach metaphysically orientated teachings with being antisocial and uncaring in the face of such challenges and interested only in their followers' own egotistical salvation. 'Escapism' and 'lack of social engagement' are the critics' favourite catchwords. Unfortunately, though, they never take the time to gain a full grasp of a teaching before attacking it. As a result they put together a hasty mish-mash of their own views and a few misunderstood concepts drawn from other teachings entirely, and then call the resulting absurdities 'criticism'.

Such misunderstandings go back a long way. Jesus himself taught this one way that leads from duality to unity – and he was not fully understood even by his own disciples (with the exception of John). Jesus called polarity 'this world' and the Oneness 'the kingdom of Heaven' or 'my Father's house' or even, quite simply, 'Father'. He stressed that his kingdom was not of this world, and taught the way to the Father. Yet all his utterances were initially interpreted in an exclusively concrete, material sense and taken to refer to this world. In chapter after chapter John's gospel bears witness to these misunderstandings. Jesus speaks of the temple that he will rebuild in three days: the disciples think he means the Jerusalem temple, when in fact he means his own body. Jesus speaks about the rebirth of the spirit with Nicodemus, yet the latter thinks he is talking about childbirth. Jesus tells the woman by the well about the water of life, yet all she can think about is drinking-water. These examples can be multiplied at will, all showing what totally different points of view Jesus and his disciples have. Jesus tries to turn people's eyes towards the meaning and importance of the Oneness, while his listeners cling feverishly and fearfully to the world of polarities. We know of not one exhortation on Jesus' part to improve the world or turn it into a paradise: instead he attempts in everything he says to encourage people to risk taking the one step that leads to salvation – that salvation that is also healing and wholeness.

To start with, though, this path always unleashes fear, for it also leads us through suffering and dread. The world can be *over-come* only by taking it upon oneself: suffering, similarly, can be done away with only by taking it upon oneself, for the world and suffering are forever one. What the esoteric teachings show us is not how to escape from the world but how to transcend it. 'Transcending the world', however, is merely another term for 'transcending polarity', and this is synonymous with giving up the I, or ego – for wholeness is attainable only when we finally stop dividing off our I from the rest of existence. Thus it is not without a certain irony that a path whose real goal is the destruction of the ego and the fusion of the self with the whole should be portrayed as a path of egotistical salvation. Moreover, the motivation for such paths of healing lies not in the hope of a 'better world' or a 'reward for the sufferings of this world' (the 'opium of the people'), but in the realisation that the material world in which we live acquires meaning only to the extent that it has a point of reference which lies outside itself.

To take an example: if we are at a school which has neither any goal nor any form of graduation, and in which pupils learn only for learning's sake, the learning itself becomes pointless. School and learning acquire purpose only when there is some point of reference which lies outside the school. Having a job or profession in view is not some form of educational escapism or 'de-schooling': on the contrary, it is only such a goal which makes it possible for pupils to apply themselves actively and purposefully to their studies. In just the same way this life and the world we live in acquire a meaningful dimension only when our goal is to transcend them. The purpose of a stairway is not to stand still on it but to use it to *rise above it.**

It is as a result of the loss of any such *meta-physical* point of reference that present-day life has come to seem pointless for so many of us, for the only point that is left for us is progress. Yet

*Or, equally, to get to the bottom of it! – tr.

29

progress knows only one goal – namely, more progress. And so it is that what should have been a way turns into a trip.

It is important for our comprehension of illness and healing to understand just what the word 'healing' means. Once we lose sight of the fact that *heal-ing* always means getting nearer to being *whole* (that is to say, nearer to oneness), what we actually try to do is seek our healing goal within polarity itself – and certain failure awaits any such attempt. At the same time, if we take what we have so far gathered about the nature of unity, together with the fact that it can be attained only through a conjunction of opposites (*coniunctio oppositorum*), and apply this understanding to the domain of brain-hemisphere theory, it soon becomes clear that, at this level at least, our goal of transcending polarity involves putting an end to the set-up whereby each half of the brain exercises dominance in turn. On the brain-level too, in other words, 'either/or' needs to become 'both/and'; while 'one-thing-after-the-other' needs to be turned into 'everything-at-once'.

In the process the real function of the *corpus callosum* becomes evident. It has to become so permeable that the two brains are transformed into one. Having the abilities of both sides of the brain simultaneously at one's disposal would, after all, be the physical equivalent of enlightenment itself. It is the same process to which we referred earlier in our horizontal model of consciousness: only when the subjective conscious mind becomes one with the objective unconscious is wholeness attained.

The universal awareness of this step leading from polarity to unity is to be found expressed again and again in countless different forms. We have already mentioned the Chinese Taoist philosophy, which refers to the two universal powers of yang and yin. The hermeticists, for their part, used to speak of the 'union of sun and moon' or the 'wedding of fire and water'. They went on to express the secret of the union of opposites in paradoxical statements such as: 'The fixed must be made flowing and the flowing fixed.' The ancient symbol that is the staff of Hermes (the caduceus) bears witness to the same law: here the twin snakes represent the polar forces which must be united by the staff itself. We come across this image again in Hindu philosophy in the form of the two polar energy-streams within the human body known as *ida* (feminine) and *pingala* (masculine), which spiral like serpents about the central canal *shushumna*. Once the yogi succeeds in drawing the serpent-power up this central canal he experiences whole-consciousness, or consciousness of the Oneness. The Kabbalist represents the same conceptual pattern in the form of the three pillars of the Tree of Life, while dialectical philosophers refer to it in terms of the concepts 'thesis', 'antithesis' and 'synthesis'. These systems have no causal connection with each other – and only a few are in any case named here – yet all of them are manifestations of a single, central, metaphysical law which has always sought to bring such systems to expression, whether on the material or on the symbolic plane. What we are concerned with here, though, is not any particular system, but simply that we should be aware in general terms of the law of polarity and its validity on all levels of the world of forms.

The polarity of our consciousness constantly faces us with two possible courses of action and forces us – unless we are determined to remain totally immersed in apathy – to *make up our minds*. There are always two possibilities, and yet we can put only one of them into effect at any one time. Consequently every time we act we leave the other pole of possibility unrealised. We have to choose – to make up our mind whether to stay at home or to go away, to work or to be idle, to conceive children or avoid conceiving them, to go after money or to forget it, to shoot our foes or to let them live. The agony of choice dogs our every footstep. There is no way in which we can avoid making choices, for 'non-action' is in itself a decision not to act, and 'not-deciding' is a decision not to decide. Since, then, we have no choice but to decide, we at least want to make the logical or right decisions, and for that we need criteria to judge by. Once we have established such criteria, the decisions become perfectly simple and straightforward: we conceive children because they ensure humanity's posterity, we shoot our enemies because they threaten our children, we eat a lot of vegetables because it is good for us, we give food to the hungry because it is the ethical thing to do. To start with, at least, this system works splendidly and makes our decisions easy: all we need to do is what is good and right. Unfortunately, however, the system of values on which we base our decisions is continually being put in doubt by other people who make totally opposite decisions over particular questions – decisions which they in turn justify on the basis of their own system of values. They go in for birth-control because there are far too many people already, they refuse to fire on the enemy because enemies are people too, they eat a lot of meat because eating meat is healthy, they let the hungry go on starving because that is their allotted destiny. Of course it is plain as a pikestaff that everybody else's criteria are wrong – and yet it is irritating that not everybody has the same criteria regarding what is good and right. And so everybody starts defending his or her own criteria, while trying to persuade as many other people as possible to share those values too. The eventual aim, of course, would have to be to convince everybody of one's own values, for only then would the world itself be good and right and whole. Unfortunately that is what *everybody* thinks. And so it is that the war about who is right gets into full swing, with everybody wanting only to do the right thing. What is wrong? – What is good? – What is evil? There are a good many who claim to know the answers. Yet they fail to agree with one another, and so we have to make up our minds all over again – this time about whom we are prepared to believe. It's enough to drive us to *dis-traction* (literally, 'pulled-apart-ness')!

The sole step that can rescue us from this dilemma is the *real-isation* that within the bounds of polarity there is no good or evil, right or wrong in any absolute, or objective sense. Every valuation is always subjective, and depends in turn on a frame of reference that is equally subjective. Every judgement depends on the observer's standpoint and personal point of view, and from that point of view it is always 'right'. Yet the world is not to be divided into what, on the one hand, 'really ought to be' and is therefore right and good, and what, on the other hand, 'really ought not to be' and therefore is to be resisted and rooted out. This dualism of irreconcilable opposites between right and wrong, good and evil, God and devil, leads us not out of polarity but only more deeply into it.

The sole solution lies in that 'third point' from which all alternatives, all possibilities, all polarities, can be seen as both 'good and right' and 'evil and wrong' at once, since they are part of the whole and consequently have a perfectly valid *raison d'être*, since without them the whole would not be complete. That is why in considering the law of polarity we have placed so much stress on the fact that each pole of existence draws its life from the other – indeed, it cannot even exist by itself. So it is that, just as breathing in depends on breathing out, good depends for its life on evil, peace on war, health on illness. Despite this, people are not to be put off: what they want is to have one pole only, while doing their utmost to resist the other. And yet whoever resists one or the other pole of the universe resists the All itself – for every part contains the whole (*pars pro toto*). It was in this sense that Jesus said, 'Whatever you do to the least of my brothers, you have done to me.'

In itself the thought is theoretically a simple one, but it comes up against a deep-rooted resistance within people, if only because turning one's way of life upside-down is a hard road to follow. If our aim is that unity which encompasses all opposites within pure undifferentiatedness, then none of us can become healthy or whole so long as we are excluding anything from our consciousness or cutting ourselves off from anything else. Every case of 'That's something I would never do!' is the surest way of keeping perfection and enlightenment firmly at bay. There is nothing in this universe that is without its justification, but a great deal whose justification cannot as yet be appreciated by individual people. In reality all human endeavour serves but one aim: to learn to see the connections more clearly ('to become more aware', as we say) – *not*, though, to alter things. There is, after all, nothing whatever to alter or improve – apart from one's own way of seeing.

Humanity has long been stuck with the illusion that through its activity – by *doing things* – the world can be altered, developed and improved. This belief is a kind of optical illusion resting entirely on a projection onto things 'out there' of one's own processes of inner change. If, for example, we read the same book several times at longish intervals, we see the contents each time with fresh eyes according to our current state of development. Were we less sure that books were 'fixed quantities', we might quite easily jump to the conclusion that the contents themselves had changed. It is with the same lack of comprehension that the terms 'evolution' and 'development' are often used. Everybody imagines that evolution is the result of events and initiatives, and fails to see that evolution is no more than the fulfilment of a constant, underlying pattern. Evolution produces nothing new, but merely makes us progressively more aware of that which has always existed. Here again, reading a book provides a good analogy: the book's contents and story are all there at once, but can only be taken in by the reader step by step. As a result of reading the book, the contents reveal themselves to the reader bit by bit, even though those same contents may have existed as a complete book for hundreds of years. The contents of the book do not come into existence through reading them; instead, as the reader peruses them, he or she takes on board what is in fact an already-existing pattern a little at a time.

It is not a matter of the world changing; instead, what happens is that people manifest within themselves different levels and aspects of the world one after the other. What wisdom, perfection and total consciousness amount to is the ability to see and recognise the whole of existence in all its validity and perfect balance. For the observer, it is being able to recognise this order of being that actually constitutes being *in good order*. The illusion of change arises as a result of the polarisation that dismembers *everything-at-once* into *one-thing-after-another* and *both/and* into *either/or*. Thus it is that the oriental philosophies call the world of polarity *maya* ('illusion') and demand of those who would strive after knowledge and liberation that they make their primary task the unmasking of the world of forms as illusory, so *real-ising* the fact of its actual non-existence. Nevertheless the step that leads to this *real-isation* has to be made within the context of the world of polarity. In the event that polarity prevents the Oneness from manifesting itself *all at once*, then it will do so of its own accord in the course of time by ensuring that each pole in turn is balanced out by its opposite. This law is called the principle of complementarity. Just as breathing out necessarily leads to breathing in, waking gives way to sleeping and vice versa, so the manifestation of the one pole brings the other into manifestation. The law of complementarity sees to it that the balance between the poles is always preserved, irrespective of what human beings may do or not do. The law of complementarity sees to it that all changes add up to changelessness. We cling to our belief that things change a great deal in the course of time, and this belief stops us from seeing that time merely throws up repetitions of the self-same pattern. The forms, admittedly, change through time, but the content remains the same.

Once we have learnt not to let our gaze be led astray by constant changes of form, we are able to remove time from our picture not only of the course of history but also of our own life-story – at which point we come to realise that all the events which we normally compartmentalise into neat, consecutive 'boxes' really amount to one and the same basic pattern. Time may reduce reality to events and happenings, but once we cancel out time from the equation we can perceive the essence that stands behind those forms into which it has 'condensed itself'. (This particular complex of ideas may not be the easiest to understand, but in it lies the basis of reincarnation therapy.)

For the purposes of our further study it is vital for us to grasp the mutual dependence of the two poles and the impossibility of hanging on to the one while abolishing the other. Yet most human activities are dedicated specifically to this impossibility. We insist on promoting health and fighting illness, on preserving peace by abolishing war, on staying alive by defeating death. It is quite striking how little doubt even several thousand years' worth of fruitless endeavour have managed to sow in people's minds about the idea. The more we attempt unilaterally to nourish the one pole, the more the opposite pole grows in secret behind the scenes. Medicine itself is a good example of this: the more we persist in striving for health, the more illness turns out to be on the increase too.

If we wish to approach this problem with a new depth of vision, then we need to learn to see through bi-polar glasses. Every time we make an observation we have to learn to look at the opposite pole at the same time. Our inner eye has to learn to *oscillate* if we are to escape from the illusion of one-sidedness to true realisation. Even though our language makes it far from easy for us to express this deep, oscillating, bi-polar view, the so-called wisdom literature has long contained texts which manage to express these fundamental laws in effective linguistic ways. Unsurpassed in his brevity and concision is Lao Tse, who in the second section of the *Tao Te Ching* puts it as follows:

> Whoever says 'beautiful'
> at the same time creates unbeautiful.
> Whoever says 'good'
> at the same time creates ungood.
> Existence predicates non-existence,
> complicated predicates simple,
> high predicates low,
> loud predicates soft,
> conditioned predicates unconditioned,
> now predicates then.
>
> Therefore the awakened one
> works without working,
> speaks without speaking.
> Within him all things
> settle into oneness.
> He creates, yet does not possess,
> perfects life,
> yet claims no success.
> Because he claims nothing
> he never suffers loss.

The Shadow

The whole of creation exists within you,
and everything that is within you also
exists within creation. There is no boundary
between you and quite nearby objects,
just as there is no distance between you
and very distant objects. All things, the
smallest and largest, the lowest and
highest, are present in you as co-equals.
A single atom contains all the earth's
elements. A single movement of spirit
encompasses all life's laws. In a single
drop of water is to be found the secret
of the boundless ocean. A single manifestation
of yourself contains all life's manifestations
whatever.

Kahlil Gibran
(retranslated from the German)

When we say the word 'I', what we are really referring to is a
complex of identifications: 'I am a man, an Englishman, the
father of a family, a teacher. I am active, dynamic, tolerant,
competent, kind to animals, a pacifist, a tea-drinker, an amateur
cook,' and so on. Basic to such identifications are decisions that
we have made at various times to choose between one or the
other of two possibilities – decisions to integrate one pole into
the identification while excluding the other. Thus, the identification 'I am active and competent' at once excludes 'I am passive
and lazy.' For the most part, too, each identification implies a
value-judgement: 'One has to be active and efficient – it is not
good to be passive and lazy.' Irrespective of how far one may try
to back up this view with arguments and theories after the
event, only from the subjective point of view does the judgement carry any real conviction.

From the objective point of view, in other words, it is only one possible way of looking at things – and a very arbitrary one, at that. What, after all, would we think of a red rose that loudly proclaimed: 'It is right and good to have red petals, but wrong and dangerous to have blue ones'? Rejecting any given manifestation is always a sign of non-identification. (That is why violets, for their part, don't reject blue petals!)

So it is that every identification, based as it is on a decision, always leaves one pole out in the cold. But all the things that we *don't* want to be, don't want to discover within ourselves, don't want to live out, don't want to admit into our identification, go to make up our 'shadow'. For rejecting one half of all possibilities, far from causing them to disappear, merely banishes them from the conscious mind's *I-dentification*.

Saying 'No' may admittedly have banished one of the poles from sight, but what it has failed to do is actually to get rid of it. Henceforth the rejected pole will live on in the shadows of our consciousness. Just as small children imagine that they can make themselves invisible by shutting their eyes, so grown adults imagine that they can rid themselves of one half of their inner reality by not looking at it. And so one pole (competence, for example) is allowed to hog the limelight of consciousness, while the opposite pole (laziness) has to stay in the dark where nobody can see it. *Not-seeing* is rapidly expanded to include *not-having*, along with the belief that the one can exist without the other.

What we mean by the 'shadow', then, (the term was originally coined by C. G. Jung) is the sum of all those rejected aspects of reality which people either cannot or will not see within themselves and of which they are therefore *un-conscious*. The shadow is our greatest threat, because it is always there even though we do not know it or recognise it. It is the shadow that sees to it that all our efforts and purposes eventually turn into their opposites. All those contents that emerge from our shadow we project onto some anonymous 'evil' in the world 'out there' because we are afraid to discover within ourselves the true source of all that is *un-holy*. Everything that we do not wish or approve of originates in our own shadow – for it is the sum of everything we do not want. However, our refusal to get to grips with this one part of reality and live it out for real is precisely what ensures that we never get what we hope for. Rather do the rejected aspects of reality force us to devote ourselves to them all the more intensively. This process takes place mainly via the medium of projection, for once we have rejected and repressed any given principle within ourselves, it continually generates fear and rejection in us all over again whenever we encounter it in the world 'out there'.

In order to make sense of these various connections, we should do well to remind ourselves once more that by 'principles' we mean archetypal aspects of being that are capable of manifesting themselves in a wide variety of concrete forms. Every concrete manifestation is thus the formal representative of a vital inner principle. Take the principle of multiplication, for example. We may come across this abstract principle expressed in an enormous number of different forms (3 times 4, 8 times 7, 49 times 348 and so on). Yet each and every one of these outwardly different formal expressions is a representative of the single principle of multiplication. Furthermore, we need to get clear in our heads that the outer world is based on exactly the same archetypal principles as the inner world. The law of resonance states that we can only ever come into contact with that with which we ourselves resonate. This consideration, which is presented in more detail in *The Challenge of Fate*, leads to the inevitable conclusion that the outer world and the inner world are identical. In hermetic philosophy this equivalence of inner and outer worlds – or of humanity and cosmos – is all wrapped up in the expression 'Microcosmos = Macrocosmos'. (In Part 2 of this book we shall once again be dealing with this problem-area, though from another point of view, in the chapter about the sense organs.)

Projection thus ensures that we use one half of all our various principles to fashion for ourselves an 'out there', simply because we are unwilling to accept them 'in here'. We said at the outset that the *I* is responsible for splitting apart the whole of existence. The *I* constellates a *you* which is experienced as being *out there*. But if the shadow consists of all those principles that the *I* has refused to integrate, then in the last resort the shadow and the 'out there' are one and the same. We always experience our shadow as being 'out there' for the simple reason that, were we to recognise it within ourselves, it would no longer be our shadow. At which point we start to resist those principles that appear to be coming at us from 'out there' no less passionately than we formerly did on the inner level. We launch ourselves into an attempt to root out these negatively experienced aspects from the very world itself. Since, however, this cannot be done – as the law of polarity makes clear – this attempt turns into a long-term project which guarantees that we shall henceforth concern ourselves most intensively with those parts of reality that we have actually rejected.

Here, then, is a law of some irony from which nobody can escape: what we concern ourselves with most is what we do not want. In the process we get so close to the principles that we have rejected that we finish up by living them out in flesh and blood! We should do well not to forget these last two sentences. Whoever rejects any principle makes it absolutely certain that he or she will go on to live it out. It is because of this law that children later take up the very behaviours that they most hated in their parents, that pacifists eventually become militants, moralists dissipated, health fanatics gravely ill.

It is a fact that nobody should overlook, then, that even rejection and resistance eventually lead to devotion and involvement. By the same token, the strict avoidance of any aspect of reality actually indicates that a person has a problem with it. The areas of experience that are most interesting and important for us are precisely those that we are currently resisting and avoiding, for these are the ones that are missing from our consciousness and making us 'un-whole'. Only those principles are capable of disturbing us 'out there' which we have failed to integrate 'in here'.

At which point it should start to become clear to us that there is in reality no 'outer' world stamping us, moulding us, influencing us or making us ill: instead, the 'outer' world acts as a mirror in which all that we ever see is ourselves – and in particular our shadow, to which we are otherwise inwardly blind. Just as we can see only a small part of our own physical body by looking at ourselves, and need a reflection in a mirror to see the many aspects that are otherwise invisible to us (colour of eyes, face, back and so on), so in just the same way we are partially blind to our own psyche, and are capable of recognising the part of it that is invisible to us (the shadow) only via its projection and reflection in the supposed environment or 'outer' world. Recognition, in short, depends on polarity.

The reflection, though, is only of any use to whatever is capable of recognising itself in the mirror. Otherwise it amounts to sheer illusion. If you look at your beautiful dark blue eyes in the mirror without realising that it is your own eyes you are looking at, you get what you deserve – illusion, rather than recognition. Those who inhabit this world without recognising that everything they perceive and experience is *none other than themselves* are entangled in a web of deception and illusion. Granted, the illusion seems astonishingly genuine and real (some would even say demonstrable). Yet it should not be forgotten that a dream, too, seems just as genuine and real while we are still in it. We have first to wake up if we are to recognise the dream as a dream. The same goes for the Grand Dream of our everyday existence. We have first to wake up if ever we are to see through the illusion.

Our shadow fills us with fear. And no wonder, in view of the fact that it consists exclusively of all those aspects of reality that we have pushed furthest away from ourselves, that we least want to live out or even so much as to discover within ourselves. The shadow is the sum of what we are most deeply convinced must be expunged from the world if ever the latter is to become good and whole. Yet exactly the contrary is actually the case: the shadow contains everything that the world – our world – most needs for its salvation and healing. The shadow makes us ill – *un-well* – because it is the very thing that is lacking for our *well-being*.

In the grail legend it is precisely this problem that is the point at issue. King Amfortas is sick – wounded by the spear of the black magician Klingsor, or in other versions by a pagan foe or even an invisible opponent. All these figures are clear symbols for Amfortas's shadow – the opponent that he cannot see. His shadow wounds him, and by himself he is unable to get well – that is, whole – again, for he does not trust himself to enquire into the real cause of his wound. This vital question, were he to tackle it, would be that of the nature of evil. Because he is not prepared to engage in this struggle his wound cannot heal. Instead, he waits for some saviour-figure with the courage to ask the healing question. Parsifal it is who is equal to this task because he goes (as his name reveals) 'through the midst' – through the midst, that is, of the polarity of good and evil – and so earns the right to pose the saving, the healing question, 'What is *amiss*, uncle?' The answer is ever the same, for Amfortas as for every patient: 'Your shadow!' In our own personal story, too, it is only the question of evil, the investigation of our own dark side, that has the power to heal. In the course of his wanderings, Parsifal has valiantly got to grips with his shadow and has descended into the darkest depths of his soul – to the point of actually cursing God. Whoever is not afraid to take this path through the darkness eventually turns into a bringer of healing, a redeemer. For this reason every mythical hero desirous of becoming both healed and healer has had to come to grips with horrors, dragons, demons and even hell itself.

It is the shadow that makes us ill – but the encounter with the shadow that makes us well! This is the key to understanding illness and healing. Every symptom is an aspect of the shadow that has precipitated itself into physicality. It is in the symptom that what we are lacking manifests itself. It is in the symptom that we live out what we are refusing to live out on the consciousness-level. Through the medium of the body the symptom makes us whole again. It is the principle of complementarity that sees to it that wholeness is always preserved in the end. If we refuse to live out a principle within our consciousness, then that principle descends into the body, where it appears as a symptom. In this way we are forced, despite everything, to live out and manifest the very principle that we have rejected. That is how the symptom makes us whole – it is the bodily substitute for what the soul lacks.

At this point, then, we can approach the old question-and-answer game of 'What's amiss?'/ 'I have this or that symptom' with new understanding. The symptom shows in stark reality what it is that the patient is lacking, for the symptom is itself the missing principle, now revealed within the body in material, visible form. No wonder that we so dislike our symptoms, when it is they that force us to express those very principles that we are most intent on not living out. And so it is that we set out on our struggle against the symptoms – totally ignoring the opportunity they offer us to use symptoms as tools of healing. It is, after all, precisely through our symptoms that we could get to know ourselves and contemplate those aspects of the psyche that we should otherwise never discover within ourselves, lying as they do within the shadow. Our bodies are mirrors of our souls – indeed, they show us what the soul can never be aware of without something to compare itself with. Yet of what use is even the best mirror if we fail to relate what we see to ourselves? It is the aim of this book to teach that form of observation that we all need if ever we are to discover our true selves through the medium of our symptoms.

The shadow makes us dishonest. We always imagine that we are merely the way we identify ourselves, or merely the way we see ourselves. It is this form of self-evaluation that is meant here by the term 'dishonesty'. As used here, it always signifies dishonesty towards ourselves (and not any kind of lying or deceitfulness to other people). All the deceptions of this world are relatively harmless compared with the one that we inflict on ourselves our whole life long. Honesty towards ourselves is one of the toughest challenges that we can face. That is why self-knowledge has immemorially been acknowledged as the most important and difficult task for those in search of Truth. Self-knowledge means discovering not the *I*, but the *self*, for the self is all-embracing, while the *I*, through its tendency to divide and define, constantly prevents us from knowing the whole that the self is. For those of us, on the other hand, who are prepared to strive to be more honest with ourselves, illness can turn into a marvellous aid along our way. For illness makes us honest! In the symptoms of our illness we live out clearly and visibly everything that we are so keen to drive far from us and so remove from sight.

Most people find it difficult to talk freely and openly about their deepest problems (even assuming that they know what they are in the first place) – yet they recount their symptoms to all and sundry in all their grisly detail. *But there is no clearer or more exact way of telling everybody else about ourselves.* Illness makes us honest, mercilessly unmasking those deep aspects of the psyche that we have long kept hidden. This (involuntary) honesty is presumably also the basis for the sympathy and devotion that people feel towards those who are ill. Honesty makes them kind – for in illness we become as we truly are. Illness compensates for all our imbalances and brings us back to our mid-point. And at this point many of our overblown ego-games and power-ploys suddenly disappear out of the window, as our various illusions are destroyed at a stroke and established life-routines are abruptly thrown into question. Honesty has its own beauty, something of which can be seen in those who are ill.

Let us sum up, then. We humans, as microcosms, are reflections of the universe and contain the sum of all principles of being within our consciousness. Our path through the world of polarities obliges us to manifest these principles that are latent within us, so that we can become progressively more aware of ourselves with their aid. But recognition demands polarity, which in turn forces us constantly to decide. Every decision splits polarity into an accepted and a rejected pole. The accepted aspect is translated into behaviour and so integrated at the conscious level. The rejected pole is banished to the shadows and compels our further attention by apparently coming back at us from 'out there'. Illness is a specific and very common expression of this general law. Under the terms of it, aspects of the shadow are precipitated into bodily form, where they are somatised as symptoms. Through the medium of the body, each symptom forces us, despite our best endeavours to the contrary, to manifest some principle that we have deliberately chosen not to live out, and so brings us back into balance. The symptom is the physical, bodily expression of whatever is lacking in our consciousness. The symptom makes us honest by making visible that which we have repressed.

Four

Good and Evil

The indwelling splendour embraces all worlds,
all creatures, good and evil. And it is the
true Oneness. How, then, can it tolerate within
itself the opposites of good and evil? In
reality there is no contradiction, for evil is
the very throne of goodness.

Baal Shem Tov

Willy nilly, we are being drawn towards a subject which is not
only one of the most difficult ones that we have to deal with as
human beings, but also one that is particularly open to misunderstandings. It would, for example, be very dangerous to
take out odd sentences or other extracts here and there from our
present account of things and to apply them in other, quite
different philosophical contexts. Again, depending on their
particular experience, the very contemplation of good and evil
can arouse particularly deep fears in those who are prone to let
emotional considerations get in the way of their understanding
and their power of discrimination. Despite all the risks, however, we intend to throw caution to the winds and pose the very
question that Amfortas avoids – namely that of the nature of
evil. For if we have discovered in illness the outworkings of the
shadow, so the latter owes its existence to our distinction
between good and evil, between right and wrong.

The shadow contains everything that we have established
as being 'evil' – and for this very reason the shadow itself has to
be 'evil', too. Consequently it seems to us as human beings to be
not only justifiable, but downright necessary on ethical and
moral grounds to fight the shadow and eradicate it wherever
and however it shows itself. Here again, though, we tend to be
so mesmerised by false logic that we fail to notice that our noble
quest comes to grief on the simple fact that eradicating evil
simply doesn't work. For this reason, then, it is well worth our

while to explore the subject of good and evil once again from what may seem to be some unusual angles.

Our very consideration of the law of polarity has led us to the conclusion that good and evil are two aspects of one and the same unity and are therefore mutually dependent on each other for their existence. Good lives on evil, and evil on good – and whoever knowingly feeds the good also unknowingly nourishes evil. Statements such as the above may at first sight sound frightening to many of us, and yet it is difficult to dispute the rightness of these conclusions, whether on theoretical or on practical grounds.

The commonly agreed attitude to good and evil within our culture is very largely determined by Christianity – that is, by the doctrinal views advanced by Christian theology. The same even goes for those who imagine that they are free of all religious ties. For this reason we propose in this book to refer to religious concepts and images in our efforts to achieve a better understanding of what good and evil mean. It is no part of our intention, though, to imply that any given theory or value actually derives from biblical ideas. It is merely that mythological stories and images are particularly well-suited to making difficult metaphysical problems more comprehensible. In no way is it incumbent on us, in other words, to refer to any given biblical story: the fact that we do so is simply the natural consequence of our received cultural standpoint. At the same time there is a bonus: such an approach exposes the specific point of misunderstanding which divides Christian theology's typical interpretation of good and evil from that which is otherwise universal among world religions.

A fruitful source of insights into our particular problem is the Old Testament's depiction of the so-called Fall in the Garden of Eden. Let us recall that the second Creation account tells how the first – androgynous – human being, Adam, is set in the midst of the Garden, where he finds himself face to face with the whole natural kingdom, and notably with the Tree of Life and the Tree of the Knowledge of Good and Evil. For our further understanding of this mythological tale it is important to notice that Adam is not a man, but an androgyne. He is a whole human being, as yet not subject to polarity, not divided up into pairs of opposites. He is still one with the whole of creation – a state of consciousness that is portrayed in terms of the picture of Paradise. Yet, although Adam the human being is still living in a state of whole-consciousness, the subject of polarity is already anticipated by the two trees.

But then the theme of division resonates right through the Creation story, for it is by a process of splitting and dividing that creation itself operates. So it is that the first Creation account already tells us exclusively of polarisations – of light and darkness, water and land, sun and moon, and so on. It is only humanity, we are told, that is made both 'male and female'. However, in the course of the story the theme of polarity enters the picture more and more. So it is that eventually Adam conceives the desire to place part of his being 'out there' and to cause it to become an independent entity on its own account. Inevitably such a step already indicates a loss of consciousness – a fact which our story indicates by having him fall asleep. God takes one side of the healthy and whole human being that is Adam, and makes of it something quite independent.

In the original Hebrew text the word which the translations render as 'rib' is *tselah* ('side'). It is related to the word *tsel* ('shadow'). The whole and healthy human being is split apart and divided into two formally distinguishable aspects called 'man' and 'woman'. Nevertheless this split has not yet penetrated right to the heart of human consciousness, for the pair are as yet unaware that they are different from each other, still dwelling as they are in the wholeness of Paradise. What the formal division does provide, though, is an opportunity for the serpent to cajole the woman (who is the receptive aspect of humanity) into believing its promise that eating of the Tree of Knowledge will grant the human race the ability to distinguish between good and evil – in other words, the power of discrimination.

The snake keeps its promise. Humanity becomes aware of polarity and able to distinguish between good and evil, between man and woman. With this step our race loses its wholeness (cosmic consciousness) and takes on polarity (the power of discrimination). Of necessity, then, it must leave behind Paradise, the Garden of Oneness, and plunge into the bi-polar world of physical forms.

Such is the story of humanity's decline from grace. As a result of this 'Fall' there is a descent from unity into polarity. The mythologies of every race and time know all about this most central theme of human existence and clothe it in similar images. Our sin consists in the *sundering* of the *one-ness*. Now the words *sin* and *sunder* are etymologically related. In Greek the true meaning of sin can be seen even more clearly: while *hamartäma* is the word for 'sin', the corresponding verb *hamartanein* means 'to miss the mark or point', 'not to hit the target', as well as 'to sin'. So 'sin' is here the inability to hit the mark, or point – yet the *point* is precisely the symbol of that unity which is humanly unattainable, for a point is defined as having location but no extension. A polar consciousness is incapable of getting the point, of homing in on the singularity that is the Oneness – that is what sin is really about. 'Sinfulness' is merely another word for *polar-ness*. And in the light of this the Christian idea of 'original sin' itself becomes easier to comprehend.

We find ourselves saddled with a polar consciousness: we are *sin-ful*. There is no particular reason for the fact in causal terms. But it is this polarity that forces us to pursue our path through the midst of the world of opposites until we have learnt and integrated everything we need in order once again to become 'perfect as the Father in heaven is perfect'. But the path through polarity inevitably involves becoming *guilt-y*. The concept of 'original sin' demonstrates particularly clearly that sin has nothing to do with people's actual behaviour. Getting this into our heads is of the greatest importance, for over the course of time the Church has distorted the concept of sin and talked people into believing that sin consists in doing wrong and can be avoided by doing good and acting rightly. But sin is not just one pole of polarity, but polarity itself. And for this reason sin is unavoidable – every human act is sinful.

This message is to be found in unadulterated form in Greek tragedy, whose central theme is that human beings must constantly decide between two possibilities, yet always finish up guilty whatever the decision taken. For the history of Christianity it was precisely the theological misunderstanding of the true nature of sin that was to prove so fateful. The constant attempt by believers to commit no sin and to avoid all evil led to the repression of those areas of behaviour designated as wrong, and so to a powerful growth of the shadow.

It is this shadow that we have to thank for the fact that Christianity was in due course to become one of the most intolerant of religions, responsible for the Inquisition, the persecution of witches and even genocide. The pole that we refuse to live out always manifests itself in the end: indeed, it generally overtakes the most noble souls precisely at the moment when they least expect it.

The polarisation of 'good' and 'evil' into opposites was also to lead in Christianity to something quite untypical of other religions – namely the setting up in opposition to each other of God and devil as the representatives of good and evil. With the devil turned into God's opponent, God was thus unwittingly drawn into the world of polarity. Yet this meant that God's power to heal was lost. God is the Oneness which unites all polarities indistinguishably within itself – 'good' and 'evil' themselves naturally included. The devil, on the other hand, is polarity, the Lord of Division or, as Jesus puts it, 'the lord of this world'. Thus it is that the devil is always kitted out with symbols of division or duality – horns, hooves, pitchforks, pentagrams with two points uppermost and so on. These are all symbolic ways of saying that the polar world is devilish – that is, sinful. And since there is no way of changing it, all the great masters teach us to leave the world behind.

It is at this point that we encounter the profound distinction between religion and social work. No true religion has ever attempted to turn the world into a paradise: instead it has taught the way that leads out of this world and into Oneness. True philosophy is well aware that in a polar world it is not possible to realise one pole in isolation: the world sees to it that each of us balances all our joys with an equal amount of suffering. It is in this sense that science, for example, could be described as 'devilish' because it stands for the development of polarity and nourishes multiplicity. Every practical application of human abilities has something 'devilish' about it, for that very application commits the energy involved to the cause of polarity and inhibits any move towards unification. That, indeed, is the point underlying Jesus' temptation in the wilderness – the fact that the devil exhorts Jesus to devote his powers solely to bringing about harmless, even useful changes.

It should be borne in mind, meanwhile, that whenever this book refers to something as 'devilish' the aim is not to turn it into some kind of bogeyman: the sole purpose is to accustom us to the idea that terms such as 'sin', 'guilt' and 'devil' are merely references to polarity, as are all the various ideas associated with them. Whatever we human beings may do, we always finish up guilty or sinful. It is vital, then, for us to learn to live with this guilt of ours if we are not to be dishonest towards ourselves. Redemption from sin means the attainment of oneness – and it is precisely those who attempt to avoid one half of reality who are incapable of attaining it. That is what makes the path to salvation so difficult – the fact that we have to pass through guilt to get there.

In the gospels this ancient misunderstanding of sin is shown up again and again. The Pharisees stand for the typical ecclesiastical view that salvation can be attained by keeping the commandments and avoiding all evil. Jesus exposes both them and their view with the words: 'Whoever among you is without sin, let him cast the first stone.' In the Sermon on the Mount he superelevates and relativises the Mosaic Law, similarly distorted as it was in his day by literalist interpretation, by remarking that a mere thought carries the same weight as its outward performance. We should note, though, that Jesus' exegesis in the Sermon on the Mount has the effect not of making the commandments stricter, but of exposing the illusion that sin can be avoided merely through recourse to polarity. Despite this, however, the people of some two thousand years ago already regarded the true doctrine as so objectionable and irritating as to try and expunge it altogether. Truth is always an irritant, no matter from whose mouth it may come. It cuts through all the illusions with which our *I* continually seeks to sustain itself. Truth is hard and penetrative, and does not easily lend itself to sentimental daydreams or moralistic self-deception.

In the words of the *Sandokai*, one of the basic Zen source-texts:

> Light and darkness
> oppose each other.
> Yet the one
> depends on the other
> as the stepping of the right leg
> on the stepping of the left.

In *The True Book of the Welling Source* we read the following 'warning against good works'. Yang Dschu says,

> Those who do good may well not do so for fame's sake; yet fame will pursue them none the less. Fame has in itself nothing to do with profit; yet profit will follow it none the less. Profit has in itself nothing to do with conflict; yet conflict will attach itself to it none the less. Therefore let the Noble One beware of doing good.

As the authors of this book, we are aware of how great a challenge we are throwing down by calling into such absolute question the fundamental demand – hitherto regarded as so soundly based – that we should do good and steer clear of evil. We are also well aware of how fear tends to increase under pressure from this theme – a fear which it is easiest to combat simply by clinging on grimly to our familiar standards. Nevertheless we owe it to ourselves to stick with the subject and to continue examining it from all angles.

It is no part of our intention to derive our various propositions from any particular religion, and yet within Christian cultural circles the misunderstanding of sin that we have just mentioned has produced a deeply-rooted sense of values to which we are all a good deal more firmly attached than we are generally prepared to admit. Other religions, too, have had – and continue to have – difficulties with this problem, if not necessarily of the same order. In the Hindu trinity of gods – Brahma, Vishnu and Shiva – the role of Destroyer falls to Shiva, who thus represents the force that opposes Brahma, the Creator. Such symbolic representations make it easier for us to recognise the necessary interplay between the forces involved. The following story, meanwhile, is told of the Buddha. A young man came to him and asked to become his pupil. The Buddha asked him, 'Have you ever stolen?' 'Never,' answered the youth. 'Then go and steal,' riposted the Buddha, 'and when you have learnt how to do it you may come back to me.'

As verse 22 of the *Shinjinmei*, the oldest and possibly most important text of Zen Buddhism, puts it, 'If the slightest idea of right and wrong remains in us, then our spirit will perish in confusion.' The despair, or distraction, which divides the polarities into opposites is evil, and yet it is the very route that we have to take to attain realisation. Our awareness needs two poles for its very operation, yet far from allowing ourselves to get bogged down in their mutual antagonism, we need to use the tension between them as a source of energy and motive power as we pursue our path towards unity. As human beings we are sinful and guilty – yet it is this very guilt, this very debt that stands to our credit, for it is the pledge that guarantees our freedom.

Clearly, then, it is vitally important for us to learn to accept our guilt without letting ourselves be crushed beneath the weight of it. Our guilt is metaphysical in nature. Thus, it is not a question of that guilt being caused by what we do; rather it is the necessity of deciding and acting the visible expression of our guilt. The autonomous nature of that guilt frees us from the fear of becoming guilty. Fear is tightness and constriction, and it is precisely this that is most likely to prevent the self-opening and self-expansion that are needed. Sin is not to be escaped by endeavouring to do good – which always involves repressing the relevant opposite pole. The attempt to flee sin by doing good leads only to dishonesty.

On the contrary, the road to oneness demands far more than merely running away or averting the eyes. It demands of us that we become ever more conscious of the polarity within everything, without shrinking from pursuing our path through the very midst of the conflict that is inherent in human nature. Only in this way shall we develop the ability to unify the opposites within ourselves. The challenge is one not of avoidance, but of redemption through experience. For this it is necessary constantly to question our fossilised systems of values, and to recognise that the secret of evil ultimately resides in the fact that it does not really exist at all.

We have already said that beyond all polarities stands that Oneness that we call 'God' or even 'the Light'. In the beginning was the Light – in the form of the all-embracing Oneness. Apart from the Light there was nothing, for otherwise the Light would not have been the All-One. Only with the move into polarity does darkness arise – and this purely and simply in order to make the Light perceptible. Thus, darkness is simply a by-product of polarity, and one that is necessary in order to make the Light visible on the level of polar consciousness. In the process, darkness becomes the servant, or facilitator, of Light – or the 'light-bearer', as Lucifer's own name reminds us. Yet if polarity disappears, darkness disappears too, for it has no independent existence. Light exists, whereas darkness does not. For this reason the much-vaunted battle between the powers of light and darkness is not a battle at all, for the outcome is already well-known. Darkness has no power over light. Light, on the other hand, immediately transforms darkness into light – which is why darkness has to avoid the light if it is not to have its non-existence unmasked for what it is.

We can pursue the operation of this law right into the context of our familiar, physical world – for 'As Above, so Below'. Let us assume, for example, that we have a light-filled room, and that outside it only darkness reigns. We can happily open the doors and windows and let the darkness in, for the darkness will not darken the room. Instead the light will turn the darkness into light. Now let us turn the analogy around: this time we have a darkened room, with light surrounding it outside. If we now open the doors and windows, the light will once again transform the darkness and fill the room with light.

Evil is a by-product of our polar consciousness, just like time and space, and serves as midwife to our perception of good – indeed, as the very womb of Light itself. For this reason evil is in no way the opposite of good: instead, it is polarity itself that is evil, or *sin*, because the world of duality has no natural limit and consequently no independent existence of its own. It leads only to despair or distraction, which in turn leads to a fresh start and the realisation that our salvation is to be found only in oneness. The same law applies to our consciousness. 'Conscious' is the word that we apply to all those human properties and aspects which lie within the light of consciousness and which we can therefore see. The shadow is the area that is not illuminated by the light of consciousness and is therefore dark – unconscious. Yet at the same time the dark aspects remain evil and fearful only so long as they stay in the dark. Merely looking at the contents of the shadow brings light into the darkness and is sufficient to make the unconscious conscious.

Looking at things is the great magic formula on our road to self-realisation. Simply looking alters the quality of that which is looked at because it brings light – consciousness – into the darkness. We are generally so keen to alter things that we find it difficult to grasp that all that is required of us is the ability to look. The highest human goal – whether we call it 'wisdom' or 'enlightenment' – consists in being able to look at everything and to realise that it is perfectly fine just as it is. This is what is meant by true self-knowledge. So long as there is anything that still disturbs us, so long as there is anything that we feel needs changing, we have simply not attained self-knowledge.

We have to learn to look at everything that exists and everything that happens in our world without letting our ego immediately get involved in considerations either of approval or of disapproval: we have to learn to contemplate with total peace of mind the whole, manifold play of *maya*. That is why the already-quoted Zen text states that the slightest idea of good or evil brings our spirit into confusion. Every value-judgement binds us to the world of forms and leads to 'clinging'. So long as we persist in this clinging, this holding on, we cannot be redeemed from suffering: just so long, consequently, do we remain sinful, unwhole, ill. So long, too, do we persist with our yearning for a better world and our constant attempts to change it. Moreover, at the same time we are caught up once again in the old mirror-illusion, convinced that it is the world itself that is imperfect, and quite unaware that it is only our vision that is imperfect and preventing us from seeing the picture as a whole.

We have to learn, then, to recognise ourselves in everything – and then to exercise true equanimity. Equanimity involves seeking out the mid-point between the polarities and then contemplating from this point the constant, alternating pulse of the poles. Equanimity is the only attitude that allows us to look at phenomena without judging them – without any impassioned response, whether positive or negative, without identifying ourselves either way. This equanimity, however, is not to be confused with the attitude commonly referred to as 'indifference' – that indifference, that mixture of uninterest and lack of commitment, which Jesus refers to when he speaks of those who are 'lukewarm'. These are people who never venture into any conflict and think that they can use repression and avoidance as tools for achieving a whole world – that same world which true seekers strive to attain through recognising the conflict that is inherent in their own nature, and through not being afraid to take on polarity consciously – that is, as a deliberate, educational policy – with a view to *overcoming* it. For such seekers know that sooner or later they have to unite the opposites that have gone to make up their egos. They are not afraid to take the necessary decisions, even though they know they will always finish up guilty in the end. Instead, they make every effort not to get bogged down.

The opposites will never unite of their own accord: we have to experience them in action before we can begin even to make them ours. Only then, when we have successfully integrated both poles, does it become possible to discover their mid-point and thence to start on the task of making them one. Escapism and asceticism are, of all approaches, the least suited to attaining this goal. Rather do we need the simple courage to confront the challenges of life consciously and without fear. The operative word here is 'consciously' – for it is only consciousness that can allow us to observe everything we do and that can ensure that we do not fail in our quest. What really matters is not so much *what* we do as how we do it. The value-judgements 'good' and 'bad' always consider *what* is done. Here that consideration is replaced by the question of *how* it is done. Are we acting consciously? Is our ego mixed up in it? Are we doing it without involving the *I*? It is the answers to these questions that will decide whether we are using our actions to shackle ourselves or to set ourselves free.

Neither commandments, laws nor morals are capable of bringing us to the goal of perfection. Being law-abiding is splendid, but it is not sufficient in itself: bear in mind that 'the devils also believe and tremble.' Outward commandments and prohibitions are valid enough all the while our consciousness is still maturing and until we have learnt to take full responsibility for ourselves. Telling small children not to play with matches is fine, but it becomes superfluous as they grow up. Once we have found our own inner law it frees us from all others. The law which is most central to each of us is the duty to discover and realise our true centre – our self – or, in other words, to become one with All That Is.

The basic tool for uniting the opposites is called *love*. The principle of love is self-opening and the letting-in of whatever was previously 'out there'. Love strives for union: it seeks fusion, not division. Love is the key to uniting the opposites because it changes *you* into *I* and *I* into *you*. Love is an un-reserved and unconditional 'yes'. Love seeks union with the entire universe – and so long as we fall short of this goal we have not yet *real-ised* love. A love that still chooses is no true love at all, for where choice divides, love does not. Love knows no jealousy, for its aim is not to possess, but to irradiate.

The symbol for this all-embracing love is God's own love for humanity. This thought can hardly be squared, though, with any suggestion of God being partial with that love. Still less would it ever occur to anybody to be jealous of God's love for somebody else. God – the Oneness – does not differentiate between good and bad; and for that very reason God *is* love. The sun sends its heat down over all and sundry: it does not distribute its rays on the basis of merit. It is only we who feel obliged to throw stones – but in that case we should not be surprised if the only people we hit are ourselves. Love knows no limits, love knows no restrictions, love transmutes. Love evil, then – and it is redeemed.

Illness is in Our Nature

An ascetic sat meditating in a cave. All at once a mouse scurried in and nibbled at his sandal. In annoyance the ascetic opened his eyes.

'Why are you disturbing me in my contemplation?'

'I am hungry,' squeaked the mouse.

'Go away, silly mouse,' lectured the ascetic. 'I am seeking oneness with God. How could you think of disturbing me?'

'How do you propose to become one with God', asked the mouse, 'if you can't even become one with me?'

All our considerations thus far should serve to impress one fact on us. We do not *become* ill: we *are* ill. This is where the great distinction lies between the view of illness presented here and that taken by conventional medicine. Medicine sees illness as an unwelcome disruption of 'normal health', and consequently not only attempts to make the 'disturbance' go away again as quickly as possible, but takes it to be its primary task increasingly to prevent illness, to the point where it is finally eradicated altogether. In contrast to this, the present book endeavours to make clear that illness is far more than a mere natural dysfunction. Indeed, it is part of a comprehensive control-system which actually serves to further our evolution. Human beings are not to be freed from illness, for the simple reason that health actually needs it as its polar opposite.

Illness is an expression of the fact that we are sinful, guilty or unwell: it is the microcosmic consequence of the Fall. Not that these terms have anything to do with the notion of punishment. Their meaning is simply that so long as we partake of polarity we also partake of guilt, illness and death. As soon as we recognise these facts for ourselves, they cease to have any negative connotations. It is only our refusal to admit them, and our insistence on judging and resisting them, that turn them into our mortal foes.

We are ill because we lack oneness. The 'healthy person'

who lacks nothing exists only in the medical textbooks. In life such cases are unknown. It may well be that there are people who for decades have developed no particular symptoms of any note or severity – yet this makes no difference to the fact that even they are ill and subject to mortality. And by 'ill' we mean incomplete, insecure, vulnerable and mortal. When one looks closely, it is quite astonishing what ails those of us who are supposedly 'healthy'. In his *Lehrbuch für psychosomatische Medizin* Bräutigam reports that 'in interviews with health workers and employees at one business concern, detailed enquiries revealed that physical and mental disorders cropped up very nearly as frequently as in a parallel sample of hospital patients.' In the same textbook Bräutigam publishes the following statistical table, based on an investigation by E. Winter in 1959:

Complaints of 200 healthy employees interviewed

	%
Irritations	43.5
Stomach complaints	37.5
Anxiety states	26.5
Frequent throat inflammations	22.0
Dizziness, fainting	17.5
Sleeplessness	17.5
Menstrual problems	15.0
Constipation	14.5
Outbreaks of sweating	14.0
Heartburn, palpitations	13.0
Headaches	13.0
Eczema	9.0
Globus hystericus (imaginary lump in throat)	5.5
Rheumatic complaints	5.5

In his book *Krankheit als Krise und Chance* Edgar Heim states: 'In the course of a fifty-year lifespan, the average adult suffers one case of life-threatening illness, twenty of serious illness and around two hundred of fairly serious illness.'

We should rid ourselves, then, of any illusion that illness can somehow be avoided or abolished. We human beings are inherently conflict-ridden and, by that very token, ill. Nature sees to it that in the course of our lives we get more and more involved with illness, to the point where it finds its ultimate consummation in death. The final goal of our bodily existence is sheer minerality. Nature decrees that every step of our life should take us nearer to that goal. Illness and death destroy our rampant delusions of grandeur and correct our every lop-sidedness.

Each of us lives from our ego, which constantly hankers after power. Every 'But what *I* want is . . .' is an expression of this urge for power. As the 'I' inflates itself more and more, it is well aware of how to press us into its service by presenting itself in newer and ever more lofty guises. The 'I' lives on delimitation and consequently is afraid of devotion, love or any move towards oneness. The 'I' makes decisions, thus bringing one pole into manifestation and projecting the resultant shadow outwards onto 'you' and the environment. Illness compensates for all these lop-sidednesses by using symptoms to force us exactly the same distance in the opposite direction as we in turn have strayed from the centre. Illness matches every step that we take in the interest of our ego's *hubris* with an equivalent step into submissiveness and helplessness. So it is that the more capable and competent we get, the more prone we become to illness.

Every attempt to 'live healthily' merely produces more illness. As the authors of this book, though, we are well aware that views such as this are currently far from respectable. After all, medicine is busily engaged in the ongoing process of developing and extending its repertory of preventive measures, while on the other hand we are witnessing a boom in 'natural, healthy living'. As an alternative to dabbling blindly in poisons this latter is undoubtedly welcome and has much to recommend it, yet it actually has no more to do with getting to grips with illness than the corresponding procedures of academic medicine. Both are based on the idea of intervening actively to prevent illness, and take the view that human beings are basically healthy and can be 'protected from illness' by one means or another. But then it is quite understandable that people should be more ready to lend a sympathetic and believing ear to such hopeful tidings than to the sobering message of this book – namely that *illness is in our nature*.

Illness goes with health as does death with life. Such words may not be comfortable, but at least everybody can check their validity for themselves by dint of a little impartial observation. It is not our aim to impose new beliefs on anybody, but merely to help those who are ready for it to become more aware, and to complement their familiar outlook with a decidedly unfamiliar one. Destroying illusions is never easy or pleasant, yet it always results in a new freedom of movement.

Life, indeed, is a constant path of dis-illusion-ment, in that one illusion after the other is stripped away from us until we can finally bear the truth. So it is, then, that those of us who are prepared to risk and tolerate the realisation that illness, morbidity and death are essential and ever-faithful life-companions eventually discover that this realisation ends not in hopelessness, but rather in the revelation that they are wise and helpful friends who will constantly help us find our true, our healing path. For unfortunately few, if any, of our human friends are so honest with us, so ready to expose our every move in the great ego-game, or so keen to make us look at our shadow. Indeed, if a friend were ever actually to venture anything of the kind, we should immediately classify him or her as an 'enemy'. But then this is exactly what happens with illness too. It is far too honest with us to excite our love.

Our vanity makes us just as blind and vulnerable as the proverbial emperor whose new clothes were woven from his own illusions. Yet our symptoms are incorruptible, and force us to be honest with ourselves. Their presence shows us just what we are lacking, what we are refusing to let come into its own, what still lies in the shadows seeking to manifest itself, and where we have become lop-sided. The symptoms show us, either by sticking to us through thick and thin or by cropping up again and again, that we have not solved the problem in question anything like so swiftly or so conclusively as we generally like to think. Illness always puts its finger on our impotence and insignificance precisely at the moment when we think we can change the course of world-events through sheer personal authority. A toothache, lumbago, flu or diarrhoea are quite sufficient to transform the conquering hero into a miserable worm. That, above all, is what we most hate about illness.

And so it comes about that the whole world is ready to devote enormous efforts to eradicating illness. Our ego, of course, does its best to cajole us into believing that everything that has just been said is a mere detail, and blinds us to the fact that the success of our various efforts merely gets us even further enmeshed in illness. We have already pointed out how neither preventive medicine nor 'healthy living' have any real prospect of success as methods of avoiding illness. What might be more promising, in fact, would be for us to reflect on a wise old proverb (always assuming that we were prepared to take it literally): namely, 'Prevention is better than cure.' For *pre-vention* means 'coming beforehand' – coming quietly of our own accord, before illness grabs us by the arm.

It is illness that ultimately makes us *heal-able*. Illness is the turning-point at which unwholeness can start to be turned into wholeness. But in order for this to happen, we have to lower our guard and instead learn to hear and see what illness has to tell us. As patients we have to listen to our inner selves and enter into communication with our symptoms if we are to learn what they have to tell us. We have to be ready mercilessly to question our own views and suppositions about ourselves, and to endeavour consciously to take on board whatever each symptom is trying to teach us in bodily form. In other words, we have to make the symptom superfluous by letting into our consciousness whatever we are lacking, for healing is always bound up with an expansion and maturing of consciousness. Given that the symptom arose in the first place because part of our shadow precipitated itself into the body and manifested itself there, healing is simply the same process in reverse: the principle behind the symptom is made conscious and so is finally released from physical existence.

Six

The Search for Causes

Our inclinations always have an astonishing gift
for disguising themselves as philosophy.

Hermann Hesse

Even now it is possible that a good many readers will be finding
what we have had to say so far somewhat less than comprehensible because it seems so difficult to square with scientific
knowledge about what causes all the various symptoms. True,
most people are quite prepared to admit that certain groups of
symptoms may be brought about to a greater or lesser extent by
psychological processes – but what about the great majority of
other illnesses whose causes have been shown quite clearly to
be physical in origin?

It is at this point that we run into a fundamental problem
posed by the way in which we human beings normally think. To
most people it has long since become second nature to interpret
all phenomena in terms of causality and to put together long
chains of events in which cause and effect stand in clear
relationship to one another. Thus, you are able to read these
lines *because* we, the authors, have written them and *because*
the publishers have published it and *because* the bookshop has
put it on sale . . . and so on. The concept of causality seems so
revealing and even compelling that the majority of people
regard it as being a necessary precondition for understanding
anything at all. As a result, we hunt everywhere for all kinds of
causes for the whole gamut of phenomena, in the hope not only
of throwing light on the relationships between them, but also of
being able to intervene actively in the causal process. What is
the reason for rising prices, for unemployment, for crime among
young people? What is the cause of earthquakes or of this or
that illness? Questions upon questions – all of them devoted
to the universal hope of eventually getting to the bottom of
things.

In fact, however, the notion of causality is nothing like as obvious or compelling as it may seem at first sight. It could even be said (and increasingly it *is* being said) that our desire to explain everything in causal terms has scattered a good deal of confusion all through the history of human thought, with consequences that are only now starting to become apparent.

Ever since Aristotle, our model of causation has been split into four distinct categories. These are identified as the *causa efficiens*, the effective cause or motive power; the *causa materialis*, the material or physical cause; the *causa formalis* or formal cause, which is the shaping force; and finally the *causa finalis* or end-cause, which is a function of the stated aim.

We can quite easily see these four causal categories in operation by looking at the classic case of building a house. As its first requirement this requires the intention to build a house (*causa finalis*); then some kind of driving force or energy, such as the investment or work-force (*causa efficiens*); next a set of building-plans (*causa formalis*); and finally further items such as cement, tiles, wood and so on (*causa materialis*). In the absence of any one of these four 'causes' the house is unlikely to get built at all.

However, because of an inner need to establish some kind of more basic 'cause', we have a tendency to simplify this fourfold picture of causality. The upshot is a pair of contrasting approaches, each facing in the opposite direction from the other. Those who favour the one direction see the ultimate 'cause of causes' in the end-purpose (*causa finalis*). Thus, in our example, the intention to build a house would be what really lies at the basis of all the other causes; or, to put it another way, the intention, or purpose, is the real cause of everything that ever happens. In terms of this, for example, what has caused us to write these lines is our intention to publish a book.

This goal-orientated understanding of causality was in due course to become the foundation of the traditional humanities, from which the sciences were starkly to differentiate themselves by adopting an energy-based conceptual model (*causa efficiens*). For observing and describing the laws of nature the imputation of some aim or purpose turned out to be too hypothetical an approach. The assumption of some kind of motive force or drive seemed to make more sense, and so science settled for an energy-based approach to causality.

To this day it is the contrast between these two models of causality that divides the humanities from the sciences and makes it difficult, if not impossible, for them to understand each other. The scientific view of causality traces its causes back into the past, whereas the goal-orientated model places its causes in the future. Put this way, this latter statement may seem disturbing to a good many people – how, after all, can the cause possibly come later in time that the effect? In actual practice, though, nobody hesitates for a moment to give voice to the idea. 'I'm off now *be-cause* my train leaves in an hour,' we say or, 'I've bought a present *be-cause* her birthday is next week.' In all such cases a future event is being treated as having *prior* effects.

If we look at what happens in our daily life, we soon come to realise that some people are happier with a view of casuality that places its causes in the past, while others are more comfortable with a future-orientated view. Thus, we are just as likely to hear, 'I'm doing my shopping today *be-cause* tomorrow is Sunday' as 'The vase fell *be-cause* she bumped into it.' Yet a dual interpretation is also far from inconceivable: thus, the reason for crockery getting broken during a domestic row could be seen either in the fact that one or the other party threw it on the floor, or that one of them wanted to annoy the other. As all these examples make clear, both views of causality are perfectly valid on their own particular levels. The energy-based version permits a mechanical approach to causal relationships, and so refers exclusively to the physical level; while the goal-orientated model concerns itself with motivations and purposes that have necessarily to be assigned a psychological origin rather than a physical one. The resulting conflict, in other words, is a particular expression of the following set of polarities:

causa efficiens – causa finalis

Past – Future

Physical – Spiritual

Body – Mind

At this point, however, we should do well to put into practical effect what we have already learnt about polarity. Trading-in the 'either/or' approach for the 'both/and' view, we should then be in a position to see that the two approaches, far from being mutually exclusive, are actually complementary. (It is astonishing how much we still have to learn from all the research into light-waves and particles!) In the present case, too, in other words, it is a question of the way I look at things, not of right and wrong. When a packet of cigarettes pops out of a cigarette-machine it is just as legitimate to attribute the phenomenon to the fact that one has just inserted a coin as to one's intention to light up in a few moments' time. (This is not just playing with words: in the absence of either wish or intention to smoke there would be no cigarette-machines in the first place.)

Both views, then, are perfectly valid and in no way mutually exclusive. Yet either view in isolation must always be incomplete, for any number of physical and energy-based causes will still fail to conjure up a cigarette-machine so long as the aim is lacking. No more does intention or purpose alone suffice to bring anything into manifestation. Here too, in other words, each pole depends on its opposite.

What may seem merely banal in the context of cigarette-machines is enough to fill whole libraries when it comes to making sense of evolution itself. Is sufficient cause for humanity's existence to be found in a past chain of physical causes, with the fact that we are here at all due entirely to accidental developments and vagaries of natural selection stretching from the hydrogen atom right through to the human brain itself? Or does this one side of causality need *intentionality* to complete the picture – an intentionality that operates on us from the future and so causes evolution to work *towards* a given goal?

For scientists this second way of approaching the problem is altogether 'too much and too hypothetical', while for those who are more spiritually inclined the first one is 'too little and too unimaginative'. Yet merely to look at evolutionary developments on a smaller and more easily examinable scale is to find ourselves constantly faced with both aspects at once. Technology simply doesn't lead to aeroplanes so long as there is no pre-existing idea of flight. No more is evolution the product of accidental decisions and developments, but the physical and biological expression of an eternal underlying pattern. Physical processes have to push from the one side, while the eventual state of affairs has to pull from the other, if anything is ever to come into existence in the middle ground between the two.

And so we come to the next problem we face in considering our theme. As a precondition for its very existence causality is dependent upon *linearity* for marking out the 'before' and 'after' on which the very idea of causal connections is based. But linearity in turn has its own precondition – namely time, *which has no existence in reality*. The reader will recall that time arises within our consciousness as a result of the polarity which obliges us to split the Oneness into a *one-thing-after-the-other-ness*. Time is a product of our consciousness which we project onto the outer world. But then we go on to imagine that time somehow exists independently of us. On top of this, we suppose that time always flows in a straight line, and in one direction only, at that. We think of time as running from the past into the future, and too easily overlook the fact that what we call the present is the point at which both past *and future* meet.

Difficult though it may at first seem to relate these various ideas to each other, the following analogy may serve to make the connections clearer. Here the flow of time is represented as a straight line, whose one end stretches towards the past and whose other end we term the future:

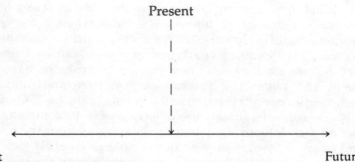

Now we know from Riemannian geometry that there is in reality no such thing as parallel lines, since as a result of the curvature of space every straight line eventually forms a circle if projected to infinity. Thus, every straight line is really a section of a circle. If we now apply this notion to the time-axis in the diagram above, we can see that the two directions which we term 'past' and 'future' eventually meet to form a circle (see diagram opposite).

To put it another way, while our lives are always based on our past, our past is in turn conditioned by our future. If we now refer our conceptions of causality to this model, the answer to our original problem immediately becomes clear: causality flows towards any given point from *both* directions, just as time itself does. Ideas such as this may well sound strange, yet they are not all that much more difficult to take on board than the familiar fact that if we fly right around the world we eventually arrive back at our point of departure, even though we have been getting further from it all the time.

In the 1920s the Russian esotericist P. D. Ouspensky referred to this time-problem in his visionary meditation on the

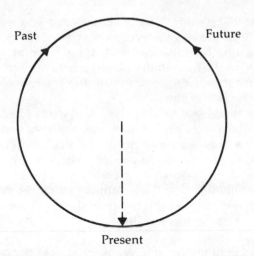

fourteenth card of the Tarot's Major Arcana ('Temperance'). He writes:

> The name of the angel is Time, said the voice. Upon its forehead is the circle that is the sign of eternity and the sign of life. In the angel's hands are two pitchers, one of gold and one of silver. One pitcher is the past, the other the future. The rainbow-stream between them is the present. You can see that it flows in both directions. This is that aspect of time that is humanly incomprehensible. People think that everything flows ceaselessly in *one* direction. They do not see how everything eternally meets up together, that the one comes out of the past and the other out of the future, and that time is a multiplicity of circles turning in different directions. Grasp this secret and learn to distinguish the contrary currents within the rainbow-stream of the present. (translated from the German version of Ouspensky's *A New Model of the Universe*)

Hermann Hesse, too, addressed himself repeatedly to the theme of time in his writings. Thus, he has the dying Klein say, 'How good it was now to realise that time did not exist. It is only by time that we are separated from what we desire.' In his story *Siddhartha*, too, Hesse deals with the theme of timelessness on many occasions...

'Have you,' he once asked him, 'have you also learnt that secret from the river – the secret that there is no time?'
A radiant smile spread over Vasudeva's face. 'Yes,

Siddhartha,' he said. 'That is surely what you mean when you say that the river is everywhere at once, at its source and at its mouth, at the waterfall, at the ferry, at the rapids, at the sea, in the mountains – everywhere at once. And that there is for it only the present, not the shadow of the past, nor the shadow of the future.'

'That is so,' said Siddhartha. 'And when I had learnt it I looked at my life, and it too was a river, and the boy Siddhartha was separated from the man Siddhartha and from the aged Siddhartha only by shadows, not by anything real. Even Siddhartha's earlier incarnations were not past, and his death and his return to Brahma not future. Nothing was, nothing will be: everything is, everything has being, everything has presence.'

As we gradually come to realise that not only time but also linearity have no existence outside our consciousness, our conceptual model of causality is of necessity totally shattered. It becomes obvious that even causality is merely one particular way in which humans think – or, as David Hume put it, 'a need of the soul'. Admittedly there is no need to see the world non-causally – but equally there is no need to interpret it in causal terms either. Here again, the point at issue is not one of right or wrong, but purely one of appropriateness or inappropriateness to the case in question.

From this latter point of view, however, it soon becomes clear that the causal approach is not appropriate nearly as often as our routine recourse to it would suggest. True, wherever we have relatively small slices of reality to deal with at the everyday level – and ones, inevitably, that are not beyond our powers of direct observation – we can get by well enough with our familiar notions. Where the scope of any given question is much wider than this, however, or where it places greater conceptual demands on us, the causal approach is more likely to lead to nonsensical conclusions than to genuine understanding. In particular, causality always needs to have a set term, or limit, to all the questioning. In the causal view of things, after all, every manifestation ultimately has a cause, and so it is not only permissible, but actually essential, to try to discover the cause of the cause, too. True it may be that this process leads us to dig out the cause of the cause of the cause ... but what it never leads to is any final conclusion. The ultimate cause of causes cannot be found. Consequently we either have to stop asking any more questions at some purely arbitrary point, or we finish up with an unanswerable question that has no more sense to it than the old one about which came first, the chicken or the egg.

What we need to be clear about, then, is that while the concept of causality may be practical enough as a tool for thought at the everyday level, it is totally inadequate and impractical as an instrument for getting to basic grips with scientific, philosophical and metaphysical relationships. The belief in causal relationships is a false one because it is based on an acceptance of linearity and time. Granted, however, that causality is one possible way of looking at things (if an incomplete one), then it is perfectly legitimate to make use of it wherever it seems useful in the context of everyday life.

Nevertheless, today's reigning view is that causality exists on its own account – indeed, is even demonstrable experimentally – and it is this particular misconception that we are most anxious to combat. As human beings, the only relationships that we are capable of observing are of the 'whenever ... then' type. But all that such observations can tell us is that two given phenomena tend to crop up at the same time and that some kind of relationship exists between them. The moment we insist on interpreting such observations *causally*, however, this last step is merely the expression of a particular philosophical view of things, and no longer has anything to do with the original measurement or observation. This dogged attachment to interpreting things causally has in fact restricted our whole view of the world and our capacity for understanding it to an extent that is truly staggering.

In the scientific sphere it was quantum physics that first saw through the causal view of the world and cast severe doubt on it. Thus, as Werner Heisenberg was to put it,

at the very small space-time level – i.e. at the level of magnitude of elementary particles – space and time are in some strange way blurred, in such a way that within such minute time-spans the very concepts *before* and *after* can no longer be properly defined. In a general sense, nothing can of course be said to have altered as far as the actual structure of space-time is concerned, but we need to recognise the possibility that experiments into what goes on at the quite small space-time level will show that certain processes can take place in the opposite order to that which causality apparently requires.

Heisenberg states his findings clearly but carefully, for as a physicist he confines his statements to what he observes. Yet these observations fit in perfectly with the view of things that has always been taught by the world's great sages. Our observations of elementary particles take place on the very borderlands of the world that is conditioned by our familiar notions of time and space – we are, as it were, amidst the very 'theatre of creation'. Here time and space, as Heisenberg puts it, are blurred. True, 'before' and 'after' become easier to distinguish as we move into the larger and coarser structures of matter. If, though, we move in the opposite direction, what starts to happen is that the clear distinction between time and space, between *before* and *after*, starts to fade, until it disappears altogether and we arrive at a point where only unity and undividedness reigns. Here there is neither time nor space: at this point the Here-and-Now reigns eternally. It is the point which contains all things, and yet it is called *no-thing*. Time and space are the two co-ordinates that determine the world of polarity, the world of illusion, of *maya*. Seeing through their non-existence is a precondition for attaining true Oneness.

In this polar world of ours, then, causality is only one of the possible ways in which our consciousness can interpret events: it is the left hemisphere's way of thinking. We have already pointed out that science's view of the world is itself that of the left hemisphere. It is hardly surprising, then, that workers in this area should have placed so much insistence on causality. Yet the right hemisphere knows nothing of causality: instead, it thinks analogically. In analogy we have a second way of seeing that is the exact polar opposite of causality. It is neither more right nor more wrong, neither better nor worse: it merely represents the necessary complement to causality's one-sidedness. Both of these are needed – causality and analogy together – to make up the system of co-ordinates which is necessary for interpreting our polar world.

Just as causality makes us aware of *horizontal* relationships, so analogy pursues the underlying principles *vertically* through all levels of manifestation. Analogy does not demand that there be any sequence of effects: instead it concentrates on the common content of a whole range of forms. If causality sees time in terms of 'before' and 'after', analogy is based on synchronicity – 'whenever ... then'. If causality leads to ever greater differentiation, analogy gathers diverse phenomena into single, all-embracing patterns.

It is science's inability to think analogically that forces it constantly to start again from scratch in each separate sphere into which it conducts research. What science is so keen to do, yet never actually succeeds in doing, is to discover some general law that it can express in an abstract form capable of being applied universally – in an analogical way. Thus, for example, it explores polarity in electricity, at the atomic level, in the acid/alkaline relationship, in the cerebral hemispheres and in a thousand other areas – but each time from scratch, and in isolation from all other applications. Analogy, by contrast, swings the whole viewpoint through ninety degrees and places all the various forms in an analogical relationship to each other by discovering a single, underlying principle within all of them. In this way the positive electrical pole, the left brain-hemisphere, the acids, the sun, the phenomenon of fire and the Chinese yang all suddenly turn out to have something in common, even though no causal connections exist between them. Their analogical kinship derives from an underlying principle which is common to all the forms listed, and which in this particular example could be called the masculine, or active principle.

This way of looking at things sees the world as made up of archetypal components, and then observes all the various patterns to which they give rise. These patterns are to be found by analogy at all levels of manifestation – as Above, so Below. Such a mode of perception has to be learnt, no less than does the causal approach. Nevertheless it goes on to reveal a whole new aspect to the world, and shows up patterns and relationships that are hidden from the causal gaze. Just as causality's preferred sphere of operations is the functional one, so analogy inclines towards the unveiling of inner kinships. Thanks to causality, the left hemisphere is capable of taking all kinds of things apart and analysing them, yet it can never grasp things as a whole. The right hemisphere, by contrast, has to forego any idea of exercising control over what goes on in the world, but at the same time it has a sense of the whole, of the *Gestalt*, and for this reason is in a position to act wisely. This wisdom, though, lies beyond all purpose or logic – or, as Lao Tse puts it:

> The wisdom that can be told
> is not the eternal wisdom.
> The name that can be named
> is not the eternal name.
> The nameless I call the beginning of heaven and earth.
> The named I call the mother of all individual things.
> Therefore the way of the nameless

leads us to see the mystery;
the way of the named
to see what is defined.
Both are one with the source,
and different only in name.
Seen as a unity, this is called the secret.
The secret that underlies this secret
is the gate of all mysteries.

Seven

The Technique of In-depth Enquiry

The whole of life consists of nothing more than materialised questions which bear within them the germs of their answers – and answers that are pregnant with questions. Anybody who sees anything else in it is a fool.

Gustav Meyrinck: *Golem*

Before getting on to the second part of this book, in which we shall be endeavouring to unlock the meaning of the more common symptoms, we should like to say something more about the technique of in-depth enquiry – the 'What lies behind it?' approach. It is not our intention to offer a book of interpretations for people merely to look up the meanings of their symptoms with either a nod or a shake of the head. To use the book in this way would be to misunderstand its point entirely. Rather is it our concern to put over a particular way of seeing and thinking, so as to enable the interested reader to see his or her own illnesses and those of other people in a quite different light.

For this, though, it is necessary first to learn certain prerequisites and techniques – for most of us are as yet unfamiliar with how to handle analogies and symbols. It is primarily with this in mind that the specific examples in Part 2 are provided. They are designed to develop in the reader the ability to see and think in just this way. Only from developing our own power of interpretation is there anything to be gained, for ready-made interpretations do no more than provide a framework which never fits any individual case exactly. Much the same applies as in dream-interpretation: books on interpreting dreams are for learning how to do it, not for looking up one's own particular dreams.

For this reason, too, Part 2 makes no claim to being exhaustive, even though every effort has been made to address as many bodily and organic conditions as possible with a view to providing the reader with the necessary basic materials for working on his or her actual symptoms. Whereas our aim thus far has been to explain the general philosophical background, this last chapter of our theoretical preamble will set out the most important considerations and rules for interpreting symptoms. It is designed as a tool which, together with a certain amount of genuine effort on the part of those who are prepared seriously to devote themselves to it, should make it possible to conduct an in-depth investigation of symptoms that is truly meaningful.

Causality in Medicine

The reason why causality is so important to our subject is that not only academic medicine, but also naturopathy, psychology and sociology are constantly competing to discover the 'true', the effective causes of disease-symptoms and to bring healing into the world by removing those causes. Thus, some seek the causes in germs and environmental pollution, others in the traumatic events of early childhood, in methods of upbringing or in working conditions. From the lead-content of the atmosphere to society itself, nothing and nobody is safe from being labelled as a cause of illness.

By contrast, we – the authors of this book – regard the quest for the causes of illness as the greatest cul-de-sac currently facing medicine and psychology. True, so long as people look for causes, they are likely to find them. Yet the very belief in causality prevents those concerned from seeing that the causes they discover are merely the products of their own expectations. In reality, all the so-called 'basic causes' are merely causes among other causes. The causal concept can only ever be taken part-way, because the search for causes always has to be broken off at some arbitrary point or other. Thus, the cause of an infection can be traced to a particular germ – but then the question arises as to why the germs only caused infection in this one case. Of course, the reason may be sought in a lowered immunity-level on the part of the body, but then this poses the further question of what the cause of this weakened immunity might itself be. One can go on playing this game for ever and a day, for even if one were to pursue the quest for causes right back to the Big Bang itself, there would then always be the question of what caused the Big Bang...

In practice, though, people prefer to call a halt to it all at some arbitrary point, and act as though this were the beginning of everything. They then take refuge in umbrella terms that are as meaningless as possible, such as 'the point of least resistance', 'inherited stress', 'constitutional weakness' or similarly ominous labels. Yet how can one justify dignifying one particular link in the chain with the title of 'basic cause'? It is sheer dishonesty for anyone to talk about a cause or speak of 'causal therapy', for the concept of causality never leads – as we have seen – to the discovery of any ultimate cause at all.

We might, though, be getting rather closer to the heart of the matter were we to base our work on the polar view of causality which we went into right at the start of our consideration of that topic. From this point of view an illness could be seen as being determined from two directions at once – by both the past and the future. On this basis it would be the eventual outcome that would actually be demanding a particular pattern of symptoms, while the effective aspect of causality (*causa efficiens*) would be responsible for coming up with the physical and bodily tools for bringing the final picture into being. Looking at things in this way would have the effect of bringing into view that second aspect of illness which is totally ignored by the normal, one-sided approach: the *intentionality* of illness and the consequent significance of the whole process. The nature of a written sentence, after all, is determined not merely by paper, ink, printing-presses, letters and so on, but also – indeed, primarily – by the ultimate intention to pass on a piece of information.

It is not all that difficult to see how reducing it all to mere physical processes and in particular to the effects of past conditioning – means that everything that is real and vital simply flies out of the window. Every phenomenon has both form and content, consists both of parts and of a whole which is more than the sum of those parts. Every phenomenon is determined by the past *and* by the future. Illness is no exception. Behind every symptom there lies a purpose, a content, which merely uses whatever possibilities are available at the time for translating itself into tangible form. Consequently an illness can take as its 'cause' absolutely any cause it likes.

It is on this fact that established medicine's *modus operandi* has hitherto come to grief. It thinks it can make illness impossible by taking away the causes, and fails to reckon with the fact that illness is quite flexible enough to find new 'causes' to justify its continued existence. The general idea is perfectly simple: if, for example, somebody is determined to build a house, they are hardly likely to be put off if somebody else takes all the bricks away – they will simply build it of wood instead. True, it might be thought that the matter could finally be settled by taking away all building materials whatsoever, but in the case of illness such an undertaking would have its problems: in order to be sure that illness had no further possible 'causes' to refer back to, it would be necessary to take away the patient's body altogether. . .

As we have already pointed out, illness has an intentionality and a goal which, in its most general and absolute sense, we have so far described as *heal-ing* – becoming whole, or one. If, however, we now differentiate illness in terms of all the various symptoms through which it expresses itself – and all of which are steps on the way towards that goal – we can investigate just what the intention and message of each symptom is, so as to discover what is the next step required of the individual concerned. This question can and must be asked of each and every symptom, without allowing ourselves to be fobbed off with references to functional causes. One can always find functional determinants – but then, by the same token, one can always find an inner meaning too.

Thus it is that the first difference between our present approach and that of its classical psychosomatic counterpart is our refusal to be selective with symptoms. We hold *every* symptom to be meaningful, and permit no exceptions. The second difference concerns our refusal to accept the model of causality that is typical of classical psychosomatic medicine, orientated as it is towards the past. To our way of thinking it is a matter of indifference whether the cause of any given disturbance is thought to lie in bacteria on the one hand or in bad mothering on the other. The psychosomatic approach has failed to free itself from the basic flaw posed by the single-pole model of causality. We are totally uninterested in past causes, for there are (as we saw earlier) just as many as we care to identify, all of them just as important and just as unimportant as each other. Rather might our approach be described in terms of 'ultimate causality' or – better – of the totally timeless concept of *analogy*.

As human beings, we are the possessors of a 'suchness', or state of being, that is quite independent of time, yet which in the course of time we need to *real-ise* and make conscious. This innermost aspect of ourselves is called the 'self'. Our human life-path is the road to this self, which is a symbol for ultimate wholeness. We need 'time' to discover this wholeness – yet it is there from the beginning. Therein precisely lies the illusion of time: we need time to discover what we already are. (Should any of this seem incomprehensible, the reader should refer back once again to the relevant analogies. In a novel, for example, the whole book is present at once – yet the reader needs time to allow the complete action to develop, notwithstanding the fact that all of it was present from the beginning.) This process is called 'evolution'. Evolution is the conscious *real-isation* of an ever-present (and thus timeless) pattern. Along the road to self-knowledge, however, difficulties and errors constantly arise: or, to put it another way, we either cannot or will not see particular pieces of the pattern. It is these unconscious aspects of ourselves that we have termed the 'shadow'. It is through our disease-symptoms that the shadow demonstrates its presence and *real-ises* itself. Neither the concept of time nor that of the past is in any way essential for grasping the meaning of any given symptom. Looking for causes in the past merely diverts our attention from the real message, because it encourages us to abandon our responsibility for ourselves and project all blame onto the supposed 'cause'.

If we look closely into a symptom's meaning, the answer reveals to us some particular aspect of our own make-up. If we delve into our past life, moreover, it goes without saying that what we find there too is no more than a variety of expressions of the self-same pattern. Not that this fact is any excuse for immediately cobbling together some chain of cause and effect: rather are both of them parallel manifestations *for their time* of a single problem-area. Thus, a child needs parents, siblings and teachers to *real*-ise its problems, whereas an adult needs a partner, children and workmates or business colleagues. It is not outer circumstances that make us ill: instead, it is we ourselves who take every opportunity to place these circumstances in the service of our illness. The patient is the one who turns conditions into preconditions.

As patients, we are perpetrator and victim rolled into one, constantly suffering from nothing more than our own unconsciousness. In no sense is this conclusion a value-judgement (it is only the 'enlightened', after all, who no longer have a shadow) but it ought at least to protect us from the delusion of perceiving ourselves as victims of circumstance, for to do so is to rob ourselves of any possibility of change. Neither bacteria nor earth-radiations cause disease: it is merely we who use them as tools for manifesting our illness. (The same observation seems a good deal more obvious on other levels. Neither paints nor canvas, for example, 'cause' a painting: it is merely we who use them as tools for bringing it into being.)

In view of all the foregoing, it will now be possible to

formulate our first important rule for undertaking the interpretation of symptoms:

Rule 1: When interpreting symptoms, ignore all apparent causal relationships at the functional level. Such things are always to be found, and nobody denies their existence. But they are no substitute for symptom-interpretation. Precisely which physiological, morphological, chemical, neural or other chains of effects have been invoked to produce the symptoms is of no relevance to arriving at an interpretation. To recognise the actual content, all that is important is *that* things are and *how* they are – not *why* they are.

The Temporal Aspect of Symptomatology

Devoid of all interest as the past may be for our enquiry, the *temporal framework* in which symptoms appear is every bit as interesting and revealing. The particular point in time at which a symptom appears can give us important information about the problem-area of which it is a manifestation. Everything that is happening at the time a symptom appears goes to make up the symptomatic context, and so needs to be taken into consideration too.

Here it is not just a matter of taking account of outer events: we need to pay particular attention to inner processes too. What thoughts, themes and fantasies were most exercising us at the time the symptom appeared? What kind of mood were we in? Was there some piece of news, some change in our life? What often emerges is that it is precisely those happenings that we normally class as meaningless and unimportant that are the truly significant ones. Because a symptom is itself a manifestation of something that is repressed, all the events connected with it are repressed too, and their significance is correspondingly played down.

Generally speaking, it is not the big things in life that are important, for by and large we manage to cope well enough with these on the conscious level. It is the small, unimportant things in life that often serve as release-valves for our repressed problem areas. Acute symptoms such as colds, nausea, diarrhoea, heartburn, headaches, injuries and so on tend to crop up at certain, very precise times. In such cases it is well worth asking ourselves just what we were doing, thinking or fantasising about at that particular moment. In trying to establish the various links, it is worth paying particularly close attention to the first idea that arises spontaneously within us, and not to be in too much of a hurry to dismiss it as irrelevant.

All this needs a certain amount of practice and a good measure of honesty with ourselves – or rather, mistrust of ourselves. Anybody who starts out with the idea that they already know what makes them tick and are therefore in a position to make snap judgements about what 'fits' and what does not will never get very far along the road that leads to self-knowledge. Those, by contrast, who start from the position that every Tom, Dick or Harry has a better idea of them than they themselves do are already well on the right road.

Rule 2: Work out the exact point in time at which each symptom appeared. Enquire into the life-situation, thoughts, fantasies, dreams, events and items of news that went to make up the symptom's temporal framework.

Analogy and the Symbolism of Symptoms

We now come to the central technique of interpretation. This is far from easy to explain in words or to teach to others. First of all it is necessary to develop an intimate relationship to language and to learn to listen consciously to what people say. Language is a marvellous tool for digging out the deeper and less obvious associations. It has its own wisdom, yet shares it only with those who have learnt to listen to it. People today tend to have a thoroughly slovenly and wilful attitude to language, and as a result they have lost touch with the true meanings of the words they use. Since language is itself subject to polarity, it too is always ambivalent, two-faced and subject to *double entendre*. Virtually all the terms we use resonate on several levels at once. Consequently we have to learn once again to approach each word simultaneously on all its various levels. Almost every sentence in the second part of this book refers to at least two such levels. Consequently if the odd sentence seems rather banal, this is a sure sign that the second level, the *double entendre*, is being overlooked. Throughout, we have endeavoured to draw attention to particular points with the aid of inverted commas, italics and hyphenations. Our endeavour ultimately stands or falls, though, on the sheer *dimensionality* of language. An ear for language can no more be taught than can an ear for music – yet both, once there, are capable of being trained.

Our whole language is psychosomatic. Virtually all the words and expressions with which we describe psychological conditions and processes are borrowed from what we have experienced with our bodies. We can never *under-stand* or *grasp* anything that we cannot physically grasp with our hands or stand on with our feet. This point leads to a line of thought which is highly pertinent to our larger discussion, but which at this point we shall merely summarise as follows: every experience and every advance we make in awareness needs to be approached via the body. It is impossible for us consciously to integrate any principle before it has worked itself out in bodily form. Our sheer corporeality involves us in an enormous commitment which often frightens us, yet without this commitment, this connection, we cannot connect to the principle itself. This, then, is yet another chain of thought leading to the conclusion that we human beings are not to be protected from illness.

However, let us return to the importance of language to our undertaking. Anybody who has learnt to listen in to the psychosomatic ambivalence of language will soon be astonished to discover that those who are ill generally spill the beans about what their psychological problems are every time they mention their physical symptoms. Here, for example, is somebody whose eyes are so bad that he can't make it all out; somebody else has a cold and it gets up her nose; another can't bend over because he is so rigid; a fourth can't swallow it all any longer; a fifth with diarrhoea can't hang in there any more; a sixth keeps turning a deaf ear; and a seventh itches because she is breaking out in a rash. In such cases there is not really very much left to interpret: all one can do is listen, nod and admit that 'illness makes us honest.' (By using classical names for diseases, academic medicine is careful to ensure that no such inner significance can be spotted through the language it uses.)

In all these cases it is the body that has to live out for real what the sufferers concerned will never trust themselves to admit. Thus, we cannot trust ourselves to admit that we are really 'breaking out in a rash' – in a hurry to break through our accustomed barriers, itching to burst out of our familiar restraints – and so the unconscious urge manifests itself in bodily form, using eczema as a symptom to make us aware of what is really going on inside us. With the eczema at our backs as a 'cause', we suddenly find the confidence to say it out loud: 'I'm breaking out in a rash!' – for at last we have found a physical alibi, and that is something that everybody takes seriously nowadays. Thus, a female employee may not trust herself to admit either to herself or to her boss that her work is 'getting up her nose' and that she needs a few days off; yet on the physical level the blocked-up nose is accepted and so brings about the desired outcome.

In addition to keeping an ear open for linguistic *double entendre*, a facility for analogical thinking is also important. *Double entendre*, after all, itself depends on analogy. Nobody would suspect, for example, that a *heartless* person might have something wrong with the organ in question. Even itching to break out of our accustomed boundaries is not something that we are particularly keen to do literally. In all such cases what we are doing is acting analogically, in that we are substituting something concrete for an abstract principle. By *heartless* we mean lacking in a particular quality whose archetypal symbolism has long caused it, by analogy, to be associated with the heart. But then the same principle can also be represented by the sun or by gold.

Analogical thinking demands a facility for abstraction, for we have to recognise within physical phenomena whatever principle they are *em-body-ing* and then to apply it to a different level. Thus in the human body, for example, it is the skin that (among other things) performs the function of 'holding in' and of delimitation vis-à-vis the environment. A person who is breaking out in a rash is itching to break through the limits and transcend them. There exists, in other words, an analogy between the skin and (for example) the various norms and standards which have the same role on the psychological level as the skin on the physical level. Equating skin with such norms does not mean, however, that they are the same, nor that there is any causal relationship between them: it is merely a way of talking about the analogical operation of the principle involved. Thus, as we shall be seeing later, accumulated toxins in the body correspond to repressed conflicts within the psyche. This analogy, though, in no way means that conflicts produce toxins, or that toxins create conflicts. What it does mean is that both of them are phenomena operating analogically on different levels.

The psyche no more 'causes' bodily symptoms than bodily processes 'cause' psychological changes. Yet any given pattern is always to be found on both levels. All psychological contents have their counterparts in the body, and vice versa. In this sense, indeed, everything is a symptom. Thin lips or a love of walking are just as symptomatic as ulcerated tonsils (compare homoeopathy's approach to patients' medical histories). What distinguishes one symptom from another is merely the subjective evaluation that we bring to bear on each of them. In the last resort it is our own rejection and resistance that turns mere symptoms into disease-symptoms. It is also the very fact that we are resisting them that reveals them to be *em-bodi-ments* of parts of our shadow – for we are perfectly happy with all those symptoms that express the conscious aspect of our psyche, and defend them as expressions of our personality.

The old argument over the precise dividing-line between sickness and health, between normal and abnormal, can be answered only on the level of subjective evaluation, if at all. If the present book addresses itself to the interpretation of physical symptoms, it is primarily in order to help those concerned to direct their gaze towards those areas which (by definition) they have not so far chosen to recognise: its aim is simply to point out that they have not yet done so. As things are in the body, so they are in the soul – as Below, so Above. There is no question of rushing in to change or cure anything. On the contrary, it pays deliberately to go along with what emerges, for a 'No' would merely force this whole area of experience back into the shadows.

Only observation can make us aware. If personal change should arise out of that increased awareness, all well and good. But any *effort* to change things will merely have the opposite effect. *Trying* to fall asleep is the surest way of preventing it; yet in the absence of all effort it happens by itself. Here 'absence of effort' represents the happy medium between trying to prevent things on the one hand and trying to impose them on the other. It is the stillness of the centre that alone makes it possible for something new to happen. Neither pursuit nor resistance can ever bring us to our goal. If, in the course of interpreting symptoms, we should get the feeling that our interpretation is in some way mischievous or negative, this impression is an index of the particular self-evaluation with which we are still saddling ourselves. Neither words nor things nor events can be good or bad, positive or negative in themselves. Evaluation is purely a product of the eye of the beholder.

For obvious reasons, then, our argument stands in considerable danger of being misunderstood, in view of the fact that disease-symptoms *em-body* all those principles that are viewed most negatively either by individuals or by society at large – principles, consequently, that are not generally lived out or even consciously perceived. Thus it is that we shall quite frequently be coming across such subjects as aggression and sexuality, because these spheres all too quickly and easily fall victim to repression as we adapt to society's norms and values, and are subsequently forced to seek expression in subtly transmuted ways. Yet to say that pure aggression is what underlies a given symptom is in no sense any kind of accusation. It is designed merely to promote awareness and acceptance of the fact. In answer to worried questioners who ask what terrible things might happen if everybody were to act accordingly, one can but point out that aggression doesn't go away merely because we refuse to look at it, and that looking at it doesn't of itself make it either bigger or worse. Indeed, all the while aggression (or any other urge) stays hidden in the shadows, it is removed from our consciousness and for that reason alone is actually highly dangerous.

By way of carrying out what is suggested here, then, we should do well to distance ourselves from all received values. Equally, we should be well advised to trade in our over-analytical and rational way of thinking for a capacity for pictorial, symbolic and analogical thought. Linguistic relationships and associations will reveal the overall pattern a good deal more readily than mere sterile reasoning. It is the skills of the right-brain hemisphere that are most needed for bringing the gist of the symptoms into the full light of day.

Rule 3: Abstract the principle from the symptomatology, and then apply this pattern on the psychological level. Thanks to language's psychosomatic nature, listening in to the way things are said will often turn out to be the key.

Enforced Consequences

Virtually all symptoms force us to make changes in behaviour which can be divided into two categories. On the one hand symptoms stop us doing what we should like to do, and on the other they make us do what we never intended to do in the first place. Thus the flu, for example, may stop us taking up an invitation and oblige us to stay in bed. A broken leg may stop us taking part in sport and make us rest. If we were to attribute reason and intentionality to illness, the behaviour thus imposed or prevented could be seen as helping to fulfil what the symptom wants of us. An enforced change in behaviour is an enforced correction, and is therefore to be taken seriously. But when we are ill, we tend to shy away so strongly from enforced changes in our life-style that we generally bring every possible means to bear on making the correction go away again so that we can continue undisturbed along our old, familiar way.

In contrast to this, it is the authors' conviction that it is actually vital that we should *let* our disturbances disturb us. A symptom only ever corrects imbalances: the overactive are forced to rest, the restless prevented from moving, the sociable cut off from all contact. The symptom forces into the open the pole that we have been failing to live out. Our reaction should be to pay more attention to it, voluntarily to do without what is denied us and willingly to go along with what is imposed upon us. Illness is always a crisis, and the purpose of every crisis is development. Any attempt to regain the state of affairs that existed before the illness struck us is either naive or stupid. The aim of illness is to lead us on to new, unknown and untrodden pastures. Only if we follow this summons consciously and of our own free will do we lend true meaning to the crisis.

Rule 4:   The twin questions 'What is the symptom stopping me from doing?' and 'What is the symptom making me do?' generally lead directly to the area of the illness's central theme.

The Common Significance of Contradictory Symptoms

In the course of discussing polarity we have already seen that behind every pair of apparent opposites there actually lies a unity. In the same way, apparently contradictory symptoms tend to revolve around a common theme. Thus, there is absolutely no contradiction involved in identifying 'letting go' as the central point at issue both in the case of constipation and in that of diarrhoea. Underlying both low and high blood-pressure we may detect an avoidance of conflict. Just as joy can express itself in tears as well as laughter, or as fear can lead either to paralysis or to panic flight, so every inner theme is capable of expressing itself in apparently contradictory symptomatic forms.

While we are on the subject, it needs to be made clear that people who live out given aspects of themselves particularly intensely are not necessarily devoid of problems in that area, nor even necessarily conscious of those aspects. Highly aggressive people are not necessarily devoid of fear, nor sexually demonstrative people without their sexual problems. Here again, a polar view is to be recommended. Extremism of any kind almost certainly means that there is a problem. The shy and the show-off both lack self-confidence. The coward and the daredevil are both afraid. Only the mid-point between the two extremes is indicative of an absence of problems. Any kind of emphasis of a particular theme reveals that there is a problem still waiting to be resolved.

A given theme or problem can express itself via a whole variety of organs and systems. There is no fixed scheme of allocation whereby a given theme has to choose any one particular symptom as its *em-bodi-ment*. It is this very flexibility of expression that is responsible for the simultaneous success and failure of our efforts to combat symptoms. Any given symptom may admittedly be overcome or even prevented, but if it is, the problem in question will simply choose another way of embodying itself – a process which is known as a *symptom-shift*. Thus the problem of being under stress, for example, can show up just as easily in the form of high blood-pressure as of high muscle-tone, raised pressure within the eye (glaucoma), abscesses or, for that matter, a tendency to pressurise other people. True, each variant has its own special characteristics, but all the symptoms listed still embody the same basic theme. Looking closely into a person's medical history from this viewpoint will soon reveal a single thread running right through it – and one, moreover, which will generally have escaped the patient's notice entirely.

Degrees of Escalation

True though it is that symptoms make us whole by embodying what is absent from our consciousness, the process cannot of itself solve the problem finally. For our consciousness remains unwhole until we have actually succeeded in integrating our shadow. The physical symptom is a necessary stage along the way, but is never the final answer. Learning, maturing, perceiving and experiencing are things that can only happen at the level of consciousness itself. Even though the body is a necessary precondition for this to occur, it must always be borne in mind that it is the psyche that ultimately has to do the perceiving and make sense of what it perceives.

Thus, for example, we feel pain exclusively in the mind, not in the body. Here, too, in other words, the body serves purely as a medium for conveying the relevant experience. (The fact that the body is in no way a prerequisite for feeling pain can be quite clearly seen in the case of phantom-limb pain – pain which amputees feel in limbs that are no longer there.) In the authors' view it is important, despite the mutual effects which *psyche* and *soma* have on each other, that we should get these two aspects clearly distinguished in our heads. To put it in visual terms, the body is the place where a process originating at a higher level reaches its lowest point and then reverses itself before climbing back up again. A falling ball, similarly, needs the resistance of some physical object if it is to bounce back up into the air. Sticking with our 'above/below' analogy, then, the processes of consciousness can likewise be seen as descending into corporeality in order to undergo a 180-degree reversal and then climb back up again into the sphere of pure consciousness.

Every archetypal principle has to become 'condensed' into bodily and material form before we can truly experience it and grasp it as human beings. Nevertheless in the very act of experiencing it we once again leave the bodily, material level behind and raise ourselves to the level of pure consciousness. Every conscious act of learning affirms the validity of the manifestation concerned and at the same time relieves it of the need to continue manifesting itself. In the specific case of illness, however, this means that problems cannot be solved on the physical level, but can only provide us with opportunities for learning.

Everything that goes on in the body provides us with experience. Just how far that experience penetrates our consciousness, though, cannot be predicted for any given individual. Here the same laws apply as in respect of any other learning-process. Thus, it is inevitable that a child will learn something, however little, from every arithmetical exercise it tackles, but it remains an open question whether, as a result, it will finally grasp the underlying mathematical principle as such. So long as the child has failed to grasp that principle, each individual exercise will tend to be a painful experience. It is only grasping the principle (the content) that can free the exercise (the form) from its painful aftertaste. By analogy, then, every symptom likewise offers both a challenge and an opportunity – the opportunity, that is, to discover and to grasp the problem that actually underlies it. Should this fail to occur (perhaps because we are still totally hooked on our projections and insist on seeing symptoms as random disturbances with purely mechanical causes), the challenges facing us will not only continue, but actually intensify. It is the resulting continuum, extending from gentle provocation at one end to severe pressure at the other, that is meant here by 'degrees of escalation'. Each stage represents an increase in the intensity with which our destiny challenges us to question our accustomed outlook and to integrate into our consciousness what has hitherto been pushed underground. The greater our resistance to this process, the more pressure the symptoms will put on us.

The table below represents a summary of this process, divided into seven degrees of escalation. This particular way of dividing things up should not, of course, be seen as an absolute or rigid system, but merely as an attempt to illustrate the idea of escalation:

1. Psychological phenomena (thoughts, wishes, fantasies)
2. Functional disturbances
3. Acute physical disturbances (inflammations, wounds, minor accidents)
4. Chronic conditions
5. Incurable processes, physical changes, cancer
6. Death (through illness or accident)
7. Congenital deformities and conditions (karma).

Before a problem shows up in the body as a symptom, it makes its presence known in the psyche as a theme, idea, wish or fantasy. The more open and receptive we are towards our unconscious impulses, and the more prepared to give them free rein, the more lively (and unorthodox) our way of life will be. If, on the other hand, we have very clear ideas and standards, then we cannot afford to admit to such impulses, for they throw into question our whole life thus far and stand all our priorities on their heads. In this case, then, we tend to lock up within ourselves the source from which those impulses generally spring and carry on living our lives in the conviction that 'such problems' are unknown to us.

This attempt to make ourselves unreceptive to our psychological side leads directly to the first degree of escalation: we get a symptom – slight, innocent, yet totally faithful. It represents an impulse's way of expressing itself despite all our efforts to the contrary. For even psychological impulses demand to be trans-muted – that is, lived out for real – in such a way as to descend into physicality. If we refuse to allow this transmutation of our own free will, then it will happen anyway, but this time via the mechanism of symptomatisation. This point clearly demon-strates the invariable rule that withdrawing recognition from an impulse results in it apparently descending on us from 'out there'.

After the functional disturbances (with which, after some initial resistance, we generally learn to live) it is above all the acute inflammatory symptoms that now make themselves felt – symptoms which can take up residence in almost any part of the body, depending on the particular problem-area involved. Lay people can easily recognise these symptoms by the suffix *-itis*. Every inflammatory condition challenges us to grasp something quite specific, and has as its object – as we shall see in more detail in Part 2 – to make visible some unconscious conflict. If it fails in this purpose (our world, after all, is hostile not only to conflict, but also to infections) the acute inflammations develop into chronic conditions (*-osis*). Those of us who fail to under-stand the urgent call for change thus receive a lasting reminder that is set to accompany them through many a long year. Slowly, though, such chronic processes tend to lead to irreversi-ble physical changes which are then referred to as 'incurable illnesses'.

Sooner or later this development leads to death. Here one could of course object that all our lives have to end in death anyway, and that death cannot therefore be counted as a 'degree of escalation' in terms of our argument. Nevertheless nobody should ignore the fact that death has a constant message for us, too, in that it reminds us in the most vivid possible way of the simple truth that the whole of material existence has a beginning and an end, and that it is therefore foolish to cling on to it. The challenge of death is constantly to *let go* – to let go of the illusion of time, to let go of the illusion of the *I*. Death *is* a symptom because it is the expression of polarity – and, like any symptom, it is amenable to healing through becoming One.

With the last stage of the escalatory process – the congenital conditions and handicaps – the end of the line finally rejoins its beginning. For whatever has not been grasped by the time of death is taken over as a problem by the consciousness into the next incarnation. Here we touch on a subject which in our culture has not yet come to be regarded as by any means a matter of course. Certainly this is not the right place to embark on a full discussion of reincarnation, yet the authors can hardly avoid mentioning what they know about reincarnation, if only because without it their representation of how illness and healing work would in certain cases not make sense. There are many, for example, for whom our basic understanding of disease-symptoms would seem to be inapplicable both to child-hood illnesses and especially to congenital conditions.

It is here that the doctrine of reincarnation can make things so much easier to understand. True, it immediately puts us in danger of seeking the 'causes' of present illness in earlier lives – an approach which is just as liable to lead us astray as looking for 'causes' in our present life. Nevertheless we have already seen that our consciousness needs the idea of linearity and time in order to appreciate what is going on at the polar level of existence. It is in this sense that the idea of 'earlier lives', too, is a necessary and sensible way of looking at our curriculum of consciousness.

An example will illustrate the general idea. A person wakes up one morning, let us say. For him (or, equally, for her) it is a new day, and he decides to arrange it as he likes. Totally unimpressed by this decision, however, the bailiff turns up at the door to demand money, even though manifestly our hero has not spent or borrowed a penny all day. Just how surprised he will be at this turn of events will depend on whether he is disposed to extend his identity to all the days, months and years that have preceded this moment, or whether he is only prepared to identify himself with the day that has just dawned. In the first case he will be neither astonished to see the bailiff, nor surprised at the physical activities or other circumstances that he encounters during the course of the new day. He will realise that he cannot simply arrange the day as he likes, because the continuity of the past extends (despite being interrupted by night-time and sleep) to include the present day. If he were to take night's interven-tion as an excuse for identifying himself solely with the new day and discarding his relationship to everything that had gone before, all the phenomena mentioned would appear to him as gross injustices designed to frustrate his purposes in the most gratuitous and arbitrary way.

If we now replace the day in this example with a person's life, and the night with death, it is easy to appreciate the difference that an acceptance or rejection of reincarnation can make to our overall view of things. The idea of reincarnation broadens our field of view, extends our range of vision and consequently makes it easier to grasp the general pattern. To use it purely in order to shift the supposed causes even further back into the past – as so often happens – would, of course, be to misuse the whole idea. But if, on the other hand, it makes us aware that this life is only a tiny section of our overall educational curriculum, it becomes much easier to make logical sense of individual people's very different initial life-situations than would be the case if every life were a one-time affair resulting from random mixtures of genetic data.

It suffices for our theme, then, to be aware that while we come into this world with a new body, we do so with an old consciousness. The state of consciousness that we bring with us is an expression of what we have learnt previously. Thus, we bring our specific problems with us and then use the new world around us to *real-ise* them and work them out. Problems do not arise in this life: they merely become visible.

Granted, problems naturally do not arise in previous lives, either, for problems do not have their origins in the world of forms at all. Problems and conflicts, like guilt and sin, are unavoidable concomitants of polarity and so are there *a priori*. In an esoteric text the authors once came across the sentence, 'Guilt is the incompleteness of the unripe fruit.' Children are just as beset with problems and conflicts as adults. As against this, however, children are generally in closer contact with their unconscious and consequently are not afraid to express impulses spontaneously as they arise – in so far as the 'clever grown-ups' will let them, that is. As we grow older, however, we distance ourselves increasingly from the unconscious and become more and more set in our ways – which is to say stuck with our personal norms and living lies – as a result of which our proneness to disease-symptoms naturally also increases with age. But then every living being that partakes of polarity is basically *un-whole* and thus, by the same token, ill.

This goes for animals as well. In animals too, in other words, the correlation between illness and the development of the shadow can be observed. The less the differentiation and the consequent subjection to polarity, the lower the vulnerability to disease. The further a living being advances in the direction of polarity – that is, of self-awareness – the more prone it becomes to illness. Human beings display the most highly developed form of self-awareness known to us, and for that reason it is we humans who experience the tension of polarity at its strongest. In consequence it is also on the human level that illness has its greatest significance.

The degrees of escalation that are characteristic of illness should give us some idea of how any given challenge from this quarter gradually increases and intensifies its pressure on us. There are no grave illnesses or accidents that suddenly descend on us out of a cloudless sky – merely people who for too long have believed in that cloudless sky in the first place. Yet those who never fall prey to illusion can never become dis-illusioned either!

Turning a Blind Eye to Ourselves

While perusing the following disease-profiles, it could prove particularly helpful to have in mind a person known to you – whether a relation or an acquaintance – who is, or has been, suffering from the particular symptom in question. This will give you the chance to test out the relevant interpretations. In such cases you will very quickly be able to judge how well the interpretations fit. At the same time you will improve your knowledge of what really makes human beings tick.

Nevertheless all this should be done only mentally. On no account should you foist on other people your interpretations of their symptoms. When it comes down to it, after all, neither the symptom nor the problem is anybody else's business, and every unsolicited remark addressed to somebody else is already an infringement of their privacy. It is for each of us to worry about our own problems: there is no greater contribution that we can make to the perfecting of the universe. If it is recommended that you test the following symptomatic profiles on other people, then, this is purely in order to allow you to check the validity of the method and of the various associated ideas. This is because if you try to do this with your own symptoms you will almost certainly find that in this one 'very special' case the interpretation does not fit – even though the exact opposite may in fact be the case.

This is where the greatest problem of our undertaking lies – our blindness to what is going on in our own backyard. The theory underlying this blindness to ourselves is actually quite easy to explain. A symptom, after all, is the embodiment of a principle that is not present in consciousness. Our interpretation identifies this principle and points out that it really is still there within us, but only as part of the shadow, where it cannot be seen. As the sufferers in question, though, we tend to compare this assertion with what we ourselves are consciously aware of, and so come to the conclusion that it really isn't there after all. We then go on to regard this as proof that in our case the interpretation 'doesn't fit'. This is completely to overlook the fact, however, that our not seeing it is precisely the problem at issue, and that it is the symptom's job to help us learn to do so! But then this demands conscious work and self-examination, and is not something that can be accomplished at a mere glance.

If one of our symptoms embodies aggression, in other words, the reason for our having this particular symptom is that we are either failing to notice the aggression within ourselves or failing to live it out at all. If we then learn about our aggression from the interpretation, we tend to defend ourselves vigorously against the very idea of it, just as we have always done – for otherwise it would never have been consigned to the shadow in the first place. It is hardly surprising, then, that we can discover no aggression within ourselves – for if we were able to see it we should not be suffering from the symptom at all. On the basis of this reciprocal relationship, in fact, it can be stated as a general rule that we can tell from the sheer strength of reaction to it just how accurate any particular interpretation is. Whenever an interpretation strikes home it tends to produce a kind of unease, a feeling of anxiety and consequently of defensiveness. It may be useful in such cases to have an honest partner or friend whom one can ask about it – one, in particular, who is brave enough to talk about the weaknesses that he or she perceives in us. It is more revealing still to listen to what our enemies and critics have to say – for they are nearly always right.

Rule 5: If the cap fits, wear it!

A Summary of the Theory

1. Human consciousness is bi-polar. On the one hand this allows us to become self-aware, but on the other hand it makes us *un-whole* and *in-complete*.

2. Illness is in our nature. Disease is the expression of our incompleteness and is unavoidable in the context of polarity.

3. Human illness *em-bodies* itself in symptoms. Symptoms are parts of our consciousness's shadow that have been precipitated into physical form.

4. Each of us as a microcosm contains within our consciousness all the principles of the macrocosm. Since, however, our

power of discrimination ensures that we only ever identify ourselves with one half of each principle, the other half is relegated to the shadows and is consequently unknown to us.

5. Any principle that is not lived out for real insists on its right to life and existence via the medium of physical symptoms. In our symptoms we are constantly forced to live out and to *real-ise* precisely those things that we least want to. This is how our symptoms make up for all our imbalances.

6. Symptoms make us honest!

7. In our symptoms we have what our consciousness lacks.

8. Healing is made possible only by making ourselves aware of those hidden aspects of ourselves that are our shadow and by integrating them. Once we have discovered what we are lacking, the symptoms become superflous.

9. The aim of healing is wholeness and oneness. We are whole the moment we finally discover our true self and become one with all that is.

10. Illness prevents us from straying from the road that leads to oneness. For that reason

ILLNESS IS A PATH TO PERFECTION.

Symptoms and their Meaning

You said,
'What is the sign of the way, O Dervish?'
    'Hear it from me,
and when you hear, reflect.
For you the sign is that,
for every forward step you make,
you will see your distress grow greater.'

Fariduddin Attar

Part Two

Symptoms and First Aid

Infection

Infection represents one of the commonest and most basic aspects of the disease-process within the human body. Most of the symptoms that present themselves in acute form are inflammations of one kind or another, from colds at one end of the spectrum, via lung infections, to cholera and smallpox at the other. In classical medical terminology it is always the ending *-itis* that reveals that an inflammatory process is at work ('colitis', 'hepatitis' and so on). In the general sphere of infectious illness, modern academic medicine has, as elsewhere, had its great success-stories, both in the discovery of antibiotics (such as penicillin) and in vaccination. If at one time most people died as the result of infections, nowadays this tends to be the exception, in today's medically better-provided countries at least. This is not to say that we suffer less infections – merely that we have good weapons at our disposal for fighting them.

If this particular form of words (perfectly normal though it is) seems somewhat 'warlike' in character, it should not be overlooked that what is involved in the inflammatory process is indeed a 'war within the body': an overwhelming force of hostile disease-agents (bacteria, viruses, toxins) threatens to become dangerous and is engaged and resisted by the body's defence-system. This conflict we experience in the form of symptoms such as swelling, reddening, pain and fever. If the body eventually gains the victory over the invading disease-agents, we have survived the infection: if the disease-agents win, the patient dies. On this basis it should be particularly easy to appreciate the analogy involved – i.e. the correspondence between inflammation and war. Here the term 'analogy' indicates that both war and inflammation demonstrate the same inner structure – even though no causal relationship exists between the two – and that the same principle is embodied within both, only on different levels of manifestation.

Our language is fully alive to these inner correspondences. The very word *in-flam-mation* already incorporates within itself the 'flames' that are so characteristic of war. (The corresponding German word *Entzündung* likewise speaks literally of the 'kindling spark' that can blow a whole powder-keg sky-high.) And with it we find ourselves in the midst of a whole complex of linguistic fire-imagery which we also use when referring to actual war. A 'smouldering' conflict 'flares up' again; we 'ignite the deadly fuse'; we finally 'put the torch to the conflict'; Europe 'goes up in flames'. With so much combustible material lying around, an explosion is bound sooner or later to ensue, as whatever has built up suddenly breaks out – a process which we can observe not merely in war, but also in our own bodies whenever a small spot or even a large abscess finally bursts and discharges itself.

For our further reflections, though, it will also be important for us to include a further level in the analogy – namely the psychological one. For human beings can explode too. Here, though, the expression refers not to some abscess, but to an emotional reaction through which an inner conflict seeks release. In what follows we shall continually be referring to these three levels at once (psyche, body and nation) so as to learn to appreciate the direct analogy that exists between conflict, inflammation and war – for it is this analogy that actually holds the key to understanding the illness in question.

As human beings, the polarity of our consciousness constantly places us in a situation of conflict, in the field of tension between two possibilities. All the time we have to *de-cide* (literally to 'cut away'), to reject one possibility, if we are ever to realise the other. So it is that we are always lacking something, always un-whole. Happy are those who are able to admit to this constant tension, who are aware of this conflict that is inherent within human nature, for most of us are inclined to assume that our unawareness of any inner conflicts means that we do not have any. It is with similar naiveté that small children imagine that they can make themselves invisible simply by closing their eyes. Yet conflicts are totally unconcerned about whether we are aware of them or not – they are there just the same. In those of us who are unwilling to work on our conflicts and gradually to work towards resolving them, those same conflicts are nevertheless precipitated into physicality and become visible in the form of inflammations. *Every infection is a conflict that has taken on physical form.* Avoiding the conflict at the psychological level (with all its agonies and risks) merely causes it to justify its existence on the physical level in the form of inflammation.

Let us consider the course of this process, then, with

reference to the three levels of inflammation, conflict and war:

1. *Stimulus*

The disease-agents invade. Either bacteria, viruses or toxins (poisons) may be involved. This invasion is dependent not so much on the presence of the disease-agents themselves – as many lay-people persist in believing – but rather on the willingness of the body to let them in. Medicine refers to this phenomenon as a 'lowered immune response'. The problem of infection is a matter not of the presence or otherwise of disease-agents – as fanatics for sterility persist in imagining – but of the extent of our ability to live with them. But then this statement applies with almost equal literalness to the consciousness-level, for here, too, what is important is not that we should be living in a 'germ-free' – that is, problem-free and conflict-free – world, but that we should be capable of *living with* the various conflicts. The fact that the immune response is psychologically influenced needs no further elaboration at this point, given the ever more definitive research into this area (into stress and so on) which even the scientific camp is nowadays conducting.

What cannot fail to impress us, however, is careful observation of this same relationship within ourselves. Those of us who are unwilling to open our consciousness to conflicts that might irritate us are forced to open our bodies to irritations instead. The disease-agents take up residence in particular weak points within the body which are known as *loci minoris resistentiae* (Latin: 'points of least resistance') and are referred to by academic medicine in terms of 'congenital or inherited weaknesses'. Those who are unable to think analogically tend at this point to get themselves entangled in an unresolvable theoretical conflict. On the one hand, academic medicine reduces the tendency of certain organs to become inflamed to mere, localised congenital weaknesses – a fact which would seem to rule out the possibility of any further interpretation. On the other hand, it has always been apparent to followers of the psychosomatic approach that certain problem-areas correlate with given organs – an idea which has brought them into conflict with academic medicine's theory of *loci minoris resistentiae*.

This apparent contradiction is soon resolved, however, once we contemplate the dispute from a third angle. The body is the visible expression of our consciousness, just as a house is the visible expression of the architect's original idea. Idea and

97

manifestation correspond to each other, just as a photograph corresponds to the negative, without actually being the same. In the same way each part of the body and each organ corresponds to a particular aspect of the psyche, a particular emotion and a particular problem-area (it is on such correspondences, for example, that the techniques of physiognomy, bioenergetics, psychological massage and so on are based). Each of us incarnates with a particular consciousness whose current state reflects the history of our learning-experience thus far. We bring with us a particular pattern of problem-areas whose challenge and summons to us to resolve them will go on to determine the course of our destiny – for 'character plus time equals destiny'. Our character is neither inherited nor environmentally determined. Instead, we 'bring it with us': it is the expression of the incarnating consciousness.

It is this state of consciousness, with its particular constellation of problems and life-tasks, which astrology, for example, attempts to determine symbolically in terms of the horoscope by assessing the precise 'time-quality' of any given instant. (See *The Challenge of Fate* for more details on this.) But to the extent that the body is an expression of the consciousness, the self-same pattern is also to be found in it too. What this means in practice is that given problem-areas will tend to find their bodily or organic counterparts in particular physical susceptibilities. It is correspondences of this type, for example, that iridology (diagnosis based on an examination of the iris of the eye) makes use of, even though without so far taking into account the possible psychological correlations too.

It is the *locus minoris resistentiae*, then, which has the job of taking over the learning process onto the physical level whenever we fail consciously to work on the psychological problem to which the organ in question corresponds. Precisely which organ corresponds to which problem is something that we shall endeavour to explain little by little in the course of this book. Awareness of these correspondences can open up for us a whole new dimension to the process of illness – a dimension which has to remain closed to all those who cannot pluck up the courage finally to let go of causal thinking.

Let us now go on to consider the course of the typical inflammation, though as yet without starting to attach any particular interpretation to its actual site. We have already seen that what happens in the first phase (*Stimulus*) is that the disease-agents invade the body. This process corresponds on the psychological level to our being challenged by a given problem. A particular impulse with which we have not yet got to grips penetrates the border-defences of our consciousness and irritates or excites us. It exacerbates or *in-flames* the tension inherent in some given polarity, which from now on we shall experience consciously as a conflict. If our psychological defences are working efficiently, the impulse cannot reach our consciousness directly – we are immune to the challenge, and consequently to all the associated experience and self-development too.

Here, as ever, the either/or of polarity continues to apply. If we lower our defences on the consciousness-level, our physical immunity is preserved: if, on the other hand, our consciousness is immune to new impulses, the body becomes receptive to germs and other disease-agents. We cannot avoid the irritation: all we can do is choose the level on which it occurs. In the martial context this first, irritative phase corresponds to the invasion of the country by enemies (the infringement of borders). Such an attack naturally directs all our military and political attention towards the enemy invaders. We become hyperactive, direct all our energies to this new problem, muster troops, mobilise, seek out allies. In short, we concentrate on the storm-centre. In the context of the body, all this activity corresponds to the exudation phase.

2. *Exudation phase*

The disease-agents have now gained a foothold and are forming an inflammation-centre. Body-fluids flow in from all sides, and we experience a swelling of the tissues and in most cases can actually feel the pressure. If we pursue our psychological conflict into this second phase, pressure and tension increase at this level too. Our whole attention is centred on the new problem; we cannot think of anything else; it pursues us day and night; we talk about nothing else; all our thoughts revolve ceaselessly about this single problem. In this way virtually all our psychological energy flows towards the problem – we literally feed the problem, blow it up out of all proportion until it confronts us like some insuperable mountain-peak. The conflict has mobilised all our psychological powers and attached them firmly to itself.

3. *Defence-reaction*

On the basis of the particular disease-agents (or 'antigens') involved, the body forms antibodies (generated in the blood and the bone-marrow). Lymphocytes and granulocytes build a wall around the disease-agents – the so-called granulocyte wall – and the macrophages start devouring them. On the physical level, in other words, the war is in full swing: the enemy is surrounded and attacked. If the conflict cannot be resolved on the local level (by a limited war), general mobilisation ensues: the whole population becomes involved in the war and dedicates its entire activity to the battle. In the body it is this situation that we experience as fever.

4. Fever

Once engaged by the defences, disease-agents are destroyed, and the poisons thus released lead to a feverish reaction. In fever the whole body responds to the local inflammation with a general rise in temperature. For every degree centigrade of fever the metabolic rate doubles – a fact which reveals the extent to which fever intensifies the defence process. (No doubt this is why folk-wisdom has it that fever is healthy.) The degree of fever thus correlates with the speed with which the illness takes its course. For this reason fever-reducing measures may confidently be restricted to extreme life-threatening situations, while all panic-attempts artificially to lower every rise in temperature should be avoided.

On the psychological level this phase of the conflict will have absorbed our entire life-energy. The similarities between physical fever and its psychological counterpart are striking enough for us actually to speak of being 'in a stew', 'in a fever of anticipation' or 'feverishly excited'. (The well-known pop-song 'Fever' likewise exploits the word's double meaning.) So it is that we become hot with rage, our heartbeat quickens, we go quite red (whether with love or with anger . . .), we sweat with excitement and quiver with tension. None of this may be particularly pleasant – but it is healthy. For it is not only fever that is healthy: grappling with our conflicts is even healthier. And yet people everywhere do their utmost to smother both fevers and conflicts at birth, even to the extent of being positively proud of their skills in suppressing them. (If only suppression were less enjoyable!)

5. Lysis (Release)

Let us assume that the body's defences have been successful: they have forced back and partially incorporated (gobbled up!)

the foreign bodies. The result is the disintegration of germs and defence-organisms alike: there are, in other words, losses on both sides. The disease-agents quit the body in modified, deactivated form. Yet the body, too, has been changed by it all, for now it not only knows all the details of the disease-agents (that is, it has acquired a 'specific immunity'), but has also had its defences trained and at the same time strengthened, too (it has acquired a 'general immunity'). Militarily this corresponds to the victory of one side over the other following losses on both sides. The victors nevertheless emerge stronger from the confrontation because they have studied their opponents, and consequently now know them and can react specifically to them in future.

6. *Death*

It may equally be, though, that it is the germs and disease-agents that emerge victorious from the confrontation – in which case death will be the result. Our treatment of this outcome as the less favourable one is purely a function of our own one-sided partisanship. Just as in football, it all depends on which team we identify with. Victory is victory, regardless of which side registers it – and even for the losers the battle is still over. Great is the rejoicing in this case, too, even if only on the other side.

7. *Chronicisation*

Should neither of the two sides manage to resolve the conflict in its favour, the result is a compromise between the disease-agents and the defenders: the germs stay in the body without actually winning (death), yet also without being overcome by the body either (healing in the sense of a *restitutio ad integrum*). The resulting picture is one of 'chronicisation'. In symptomatic terms this state of affairs expresses itself in a permanently raised count of lympho- and granulocytes and of antibodies, in slightly higher blood sedimentation and in marginally raised temperature. The failure to clear up the situation produces a disease-focus within the body which from now on will constantly absorb energy at the expense of the rest of the organism: the patient feels run down, tired, lacking in drive, listless, apathetic. He or she is not exactly ill, yet not exactly well either – no proper war and no proper peace, but just a compromise – and consequently is *lazy*, like all life's compromises. Compromise is the last refuge of cowards, of the 'lukewarm' (Jesus says, 'I would you were hot or cold. But because you are lukewarm, and neither hot nor cold, I will spew you out of my mouth.'), who go in constant fear of the consequences of their acts and of the responsibility which those acts consequently lay on their shoulders. Yet compromise is never a solution, for it neither represents the absolute balance between the two opposing poles, nor has it the power to unify. Compromise spells long-lasting discord and consequent stagnation. Militarily it corresponds to trench-warfare (as in the First World War), and this goes on using up energy and raw materials until all the other areas of the economy, the culture and so on are significantly weakened and incapacitated.

In the psychological context it is chronicisation that corresponds to trench-warfare. We get irretrievably enmeshed in the conflict and can find neither the will nor the energy to come to any decision. Every decision costs sacrifices – at any given moment, after all, we can only do this *or* that – and this necessity of sacrifice fills us with dread. So it is that many of us freeze rigid in the midst of our conflicts, incapable of helping either of the two poles to victory. We spend all our time weighing up which decision is right and which wrong, without realising that right and wrong do not exist in the abstract at all. In any case, in order to become whole we need *both* poles. Yet within the context of polarity we cannot *real-ise* both of them at once, but only one after the other. So let us at least begin with one of them – and *de-cide*!

Every decision is a liberation. Chronic trench-warfare merely goes on soaking up energy; on the psychological level, similarly, it leads only to listlessness, lack of drive and ultimately resignation. As soon as we win through to one pole or other of the conflict, however, we quickly become aware of all the energy that this releases. Just as the body emerges strengthened from infection, so the psyche, too, comes out stronger from each conflict for, by dint of getting to grips with the problem, it has succeeded in learning, has extended its boundaries as a result of its dealings with the two opposing poles and has consequently become more aware. From every conflict we undergo we gain specific information (self-awareness) which, just like our human 'specific immunity', will enable us to cope safely with the same problem in future.

What is more, each conflict we live through also teaches us to cope better and more confidently with conflicts in general – a phenomenon which corresponds to the body's *general* immunity.

Just as on the physical level every resolution demands high sacrifices, especially of the opposite side, so each decision on the psyche's part involves plenty of sacrifices too; for so many former views and opinions, so many dearly-held attitudes and familiar ways have to be consigned to the grave. Yet everything new presupposes the death of the old. And so it comes about that, just as the larger inflammation-sites often leave scars behind them, so in the psyche, too, scars often remain, which we then look back on in retrospect as memories of fundamental turning-points in our lives.

Time was when all parents knew that when a child survives a children's illness (all 'children's illnesses' are infectious illnesses) it takes a step forward in development or maturity. After the illness the child is no longer the same as before. The illness has brought about a change that has made it more mature. But then it is not only childhood illnesses that have such a maturing effect. Just as the body itself emerges strengthened from each infectious illness that it survives, so the whole human being comes out of each conflict with greater maturity. For it is only challenges that make us strong and fit. All the world's high cultures arose as a result of the severest challenges, and Darwin himself traced back the development of the various species to their success in mastering environmental conditions (an aspect of Darwinism which at the same time is by no means universally accepted!).

'War is the father of all things,' says Heraclitus, and anybody who understands the statement in its true sense is well aware that this claim represents one of the most basic pieces of wisdom. It is war, conflict, the tension between the poles that release life's energies and alone assure progress and development – dangerous and liable to misunderstanding though such assertions may seem at a time when the wolves have put on sheep's clothing and taken to presenting their repressed aggression as a love of peace.

We have deliberately compared the development of inflammation step by step with what happens in actual warfare because this can lend our argument a vividness which will perhaps discourage the reader from passing over what we have said too quickly, or with a mere approving nod of the head. We are living in an era and a culture which are opposed to conflict to an extreme degree. At all levels people are currently doing their utmost to avoid conflict – yet without realising that this attitude actually works against the development of awareness. Admittedly, in a polar world it is always possible for us to take various practical steps to avoid particular conflicts, but these very attempts merely cause them to break out in other spheres in more and more complex transmutations that hardly anybody has even started to take account of as yet.

Our current theme – infectious illness – is a good case in point. True, in our presentation thus far we have looked at the structure of conflict and that of inflammation in tandem in order to establish how much they have in common – yet in actual human beings the two of them seldom, if ever, run concurrently. Instead, what tends to happen is that the one aspect replaces the other on an either/or basis. If an impulse succeeds in penetrating the psyche's defences and thus in making us aware of the conflict in question, the already-outlined process whereby we come to grips with conflict takes place purely within the psyche, and as a rule no bodily infection results. If, on the other hand, we refuse to open ourselves to the conflict, resisting everything that might undermine the artificially maintained integrity of our familiar world, the conflict descends into the body, where it has to be lived out as an inflammation on the physical level.

Inflammation is conflict transferred onto the physical level. But this fact should not cause us to make the mistake of looking at our infectious illnesses purely superficially and to conclude from them that we 'don't have any inner conflicts after all'. It is precisely this refusal to recognise our own inner conflict that leads to illness. If we really want to investigate what is going on we need to take far more pains over it than a mere passing glance. What is needed is a devastating honesty that causes the psyche no less discomfort – no less 'pains' – than infection causes the body. But it is precisely this discomfort – this *pain-ful-ness* – that we are always so anxious to avoid.

Granted, conflicts always hurt. Regardless of what level we experience them on – be it war, inner conflict or illness – they are never nice. But then considerations of 'nice' or 'not nice' are no basis for our present argument, for once we have admitted that we cannot avoid any of it, the question no longer even poses itself. In those of us who refuse to allow ourselves to explode psychologically, *it* explodes physically (in the form of an abscess). How, then, can there be any question of 'nicer' or 'better'? Illness, truly, makes us honest!

Yet when it comes down to it, all the highly praised efforts of our times to avoid problems on whatever level are honest too. In view of what we have already said, even our so far successful efforts to fight infectious diseases can be seen in a new light. The fight against infections is the fight against conflicts on the physical level. And here the name given to the chief weapon involved is certainly honest – antibiotics. This word is composed of the two Greek words *anti* (against) and *bios* (life). Antibiotics are thus 'substances that are directed against life'. What honesty!

This 'hostility to life' that is characteristic of antibiotics fits the case on two levels. If we recall that conflict is actually the very engine of development – of life itself – then the repression of any conflict is at the same time an attack on the life-dynamic too.

Yet antibiotics are also hostile to life in the narrower, medical sense. Inflammations represent an acute – that is, both rapid and immediate – clearing up of problems, as a result of which toxins are expelled from the body via suppuration (pus-formation). If such clearing-up processes are neutralised repeatedly and in the long term, the hostile toxins have to be stored up in the body (mostly within the connective tissue), where their degenerating effects can lead to an increased capacity for cancerous developments. What we have here, then, is a case of the 'dustbin-effect'. We can either empty the dustbin regularly (infection) or keep on gathering rubbish until the whole house is endangered by the rubbish's own life-forms (cancer). Antibiotics are foreign substances which sufferers have not produced by their own efforts, and which consequently deceive them about what the real fruits of their illness are – the fruits of learning that are to be gathered from actually coming to grips with the problems involved.

At this point the subject of vaccination also deserves to be considered briefly from the same angle. There are two basic forms of vaccination – namely 'active' and 'passive' immunisation. In passive immunisation what is administered is antibodies that have been produced inside other organisms. It is to this form of vaccination that we resort when a disease has already struck (tetanus antiserum for fighting tetanus germs, for example). On the psychological level this would correspond to taking on board ready-made solutions, commandments and moral precepts. Either way, we get involved in patent remedies and thus avoid getting to grips with the problem ourselves or learning from the experience – a convenient way that is actually no way at all, since it doesn't get us anywhere.

In active immunisation, by contrast, weakened (disarmed) germs are administered so that the body can manufacture its own antibodies in response to this stimulus. Into this category fall all the preventive vaccines such as oral polio vaccine, smallpox vaccine, tetanus toxoid for preventing tetanus and so on. This approach corresponds in the psychological context to working out trouble-shooting techniques in harmless situations (the counterpart of military manoeuvres). A good many pedagogical efforts and also most group-therapies fall into this category. The idea here is to learn and to take on board conflict-resolving strategies in protected situations so as to permit people to cope with real conflicts with greater awareness.

None of these reflections should be misinterpreted as prescriptions. It is not a question of whether one should have oneself vaccinated or not, or of whether antibiotics should never be used. In the final analysis what we do is a matter of total indifference – so long as we *know* what we are doing! What we are concerned with here is awareness, not ready-made commandments or prohibitions.

The question remains, though, whether the physical disease-process is in itself in any position to replace the psychological process. This question is none too easy to answer, in view of the fact that our mental division of *psyche* from *soma* is only a theoretical device and is not something that we actually encounter anything like so clearly in practice. For whatever goes on in the body we always experience in our consciousness – in the psyche – too. If we hit ourselves on the thumb with a hammer, we say 'My thumb hurts.' But this is not entirely accurate, since the pain occurs exclusively in the mind, not in the thumb. The 'pain' is merely a psychological perception which we project into the thumb.

It is precisely because pain is a psychological phenomenon that we are able to exercise so much influence over it – through diversion, hypnosis, narcosis, acupuncture and so on. (We would invite anybody who thinks this point overdone to recall once again the phenomenon of phantom-limb pain!) Everything we experience and suffer in the course of the physical disease-process occurs exclusively in our consciousness. The distinction between 'psychological' and 'somatic' refers solely to the particular screen onto which we project it. People who are love-sick project their perceptions onto something non-physical – namely love – whereas sufferers from angina project what they perceive onto the throat: yet both are suffering purely in the mind. Matter – including the body – can only ever serve as a projection-screen: in itself it is never a place where problems can be resolved. As a projection-screen the body can represent an ideal aid to better recognition, yet the solution can only ever be discovered by consciousness itself. So it is that the process of every physical illness represents the symbolic working-out of a particular problem whose educational fruits bid fair to enrich our consciousness. This is also the reason why every illness that we survive brings in its train a further step towards maturity.

And so there arises a rhythm between the physical and the psychological treatment of each problem. If the problem proves incapable of being resolved purely at the consciousness-level, the body is called in as a material aid for dramatising the unresolved problem in symbolic form. The lessons learnt from this are then referred back to the psyche once the illness has been successfully survived. If, however, the psyche is still unable to grasp what is involved despite all the newly gained experiences, the problem descends all over again onto the physical level so that further practical experiences can be gathered. (It is no accident that terms such as 'grasp' and 'under-stand' designate quite specific body-attitudes!) This exchange is repeated for as long as it takes for the experiences gained to enable the consciousness finally to resolve the problem or conflict in question.

This procedure can be illustrated graphically in the following way. A pupil (let us say) has to learn mental arithmetic. So we give him (or her) an exercise to do (i.e. a problem). If he cannot do it in his head, we put a notebook (something physical) in his hand as an aid. Now he projects the problem onto the notebook and by this means (as well as in his head) is able to solve it. Next we give him a further exercise to do without the notebook. If he cannot do it, he gets the physical aid back again – and this goes on until he is able to do without the notebook because he has finally learnt to do the calculations in his head, without any material aid. In the last resort, after all, calculations are always done in the head, never on paper – but projecting the problem onto the visible level makes the learning process easier.

If we have made the point at such length, it is because a true grasp of this particular relationship between body and psyche leads to a conclusion which is actually far from obvious: namely that the body is not the place for resolving our problems at all. Yet this is precisely the route followed by the whole of academic medicine. Its devotees all gaze in fascination at what is happening to the body, and attempt all the time to resolve illness at the physical level.

Yet at this level there is nothing whatever to resolve. Any attempt to do so is rather like remodelling the notebook every time our pupil has problems finding the answer. Being human is something which takes place at the consciousness-level and is merely mirrored in the body. Constantly polishing the mirror makes no difference to whoever is reflected in it. (Would that it were so simple!) We need to stop looking in the mirror for the cause and solution of all our reflected problems: instead we should use the mirror to get to know ourselves.

INFECTION = A CONFLICT MADE FLESH

Those who are prone to inflammations are attempting to avoid conflicts.

In the case of an infectious illness, ask yourself the following questions:

1. What conflict in my life am I failing to see?
2. What conflict am I dodging?
3. What conflict am I failing to admit to?

To establish just what the conflict is about, take careful note of the symbolism of the affected organ or part of the body.

Two

Resistance

To resist is *not to let in*. The opposite of resistance is love. Love can be defined from a whole variety of angles and on a whole variety of levels, yet all forms of love can be reduced to *the act of letting in*. In love we open up our frontiers and let in something which formerly lay beyond those frontiers. We generally call this frontier *I* (or 'ego') and treat everything that lies outside that personal identity as *you* ('not-I'). In love this frontier is opened up to allow in the 'you' so that it, too, can become one with the 'I'. Wherever we set up frontiers we lack love: wherever we let something in we are expressing love. Ever since Freud we have used the term 'defence mechanisms' for the various ploys which our conscious mind uses to prevent any invasion of threatening contents from the subconscious.

At this point it is important for us once again not to lose sight of the equation *microsomos = macrocosmos*, for every rejection of and resistance to any manifestation from outside is always an expression of some inner, psychological resistance. Every resistance strengthens our ego, for it helps to establish our frontiers. That is why we always find saying 'No' so much more gratifying than saying 'Yes'. Every 'no', every resistance, makes us aware of our frontiers, of our 'I', whereas every time we go along with something those frontiers become blurred and indistinct – and in the process we lose sight of ourselves. It is no mean task to demonstrate in print exactly what is meant by the term 'defence-mechanisms', because whatever we manage to describe is at best likely to be attributed to other people. Suffice it to say that our defence-mechanisms are the sum of what stands in the way of our becoming whole and complete. In theory the path to enlightenment is quite simple to formulate: everything that is, is good. Go along with everything that is, and we become one with everything that is. This is the way of love.

Every 'Yes, but...' that arises at this point is a form of resistance that gets in the way of our becoming One. And with this begin all the various colourful games of the ego, which does not hesitate to place in the service of its self-definition the most pious, the most clever, even the most noble of theories. And so it is that we go on to play out the game of life.

The more quick-witted among us may of course object that if everything that is, is good, resistance must be good too! True enough – so it is, for in a polar world our consequent awareness of so much friction furthers our development. Yet in the last resort it is merely a device which we make redundant in the very act of using it. By the same token illness, too, is perfectly valid – and we are keen just the same to transmute it into healing.

Just as we turn our psychological resistance against the contents of our consciousness on the inner level – contents that have become classified as 'dangerous' and therefore have to be prevented from emerging into the conscious mind – so our bodily resistance is directed against those outer foes that are known as 'germs' or 'toxins'. At the same time we are so confident in handling the system of values that we have cobbled together for ourselves that we imagine for the most part that these criteria are somehow absolute. Yet there are no foes other than those that we ourselves have designated as such. (It is instructive, for example, to look at all the fun that the various dietary gurus have with identifying 'enemies'. Here there is next to nothing that is not labelled by one system or the other as dreadfully harmful, at the very same time as its rivals, in flat contradiction, are recommending it as entirely healthy. For our part, we would particularly recommend the following diet: read all the diet-books very thoroughly – then eat whatever you like.) There are some people, indeed, whose originality in finding 'hostile' entities is so striking that we go so far as to label them as ill – and here we are referring to those who suffer from allergies.

Allergies

An allergy is an over-reaction to some substance that is regarded as hostile. In the context of the body's survival-mechanisms this built-in defence-reaction is entirely valid. The body's immune-system forms antibodies against the allergens and thus corresponds to a bodily defence-reaction against hostile invaders which, from the body's point of view, is perfectly reasonable. In those who are allergic, however, this inherently sensible defence-reaction is exaggerated out of all proportion. They build up a high level of defences, while extending the 'hostile' category to cover an ever greater area. More and more substances are identified as 'enemies', and the defence armoury is therefore increasingly strengthened in order to counter this host of enemies effectively. However, just as a high level of armaments in the military field always signifies a high level of aggression, so allergies are a sign of strong resistance and aggression that have been repressed into bodily form. Those who are allergic have problems with their aggression, which they do not recognise and consequently for the most part do not live out either.

(In order to avoid any misunderstandings at this point we would recall the reader's attention to the fact that we speak of a 'repressed' aspect of the psyche when those concerned are not consciously aware of it as such. It may very well be that they are living out that aspect – yet they are still unaware of it. On the other hand it may be that the same aspect is so rigorously repressed that they are not living it out at all. Consequently an aggressive person is just as likely as a totally gentle person to be one who has repressed his or her aggression!)

What has happened in the case of an allergy is that the aggression has precipitated itself out of the psyche and into the body, and is now giving vent to itself at this new level, where the patients concerned can defend and attack, fight and conquer it to their hearts' content. So as not to bring this jolly pastime to a premature end for lack of enemies, quite harmless things are turned into enemies. Flower pollen, cat fur, horsehair, dust, detergents, smoke, strawberries, dogs or tomatoes – the choice is endless, for allergy sufferers will draw the line at nothing. If need be, they will come to blows with anything and everything, though generally they prefer particular favourites that are especially heavy with symbolism.

It is well known how closely aggression is always bound up with fear. We only ever attack what we are afraid of. By looking closely at the preferred allergens in any given case we can generally find out quite readily which areas of life it is that are striking so much fear into the allergy sufferer, and which he or she consequently finds it necessary to fight symbolically with such ardour. Foremost among these is the hair of domestic pets, and above all cat fur. People associate cat fur (indeed, fur generally) with stroking and petting – it is soft and cosy, snuggly and nevertheless 'animal'. It symbolises love, and has a sexual connotation (compare, for example, the cuddly toys that children take to bed with them). Much the same applies to rabbit fur. In horses the instinctive, animal element is more to the fore, in dogs the aggressive aspect – yet these are fine distinctions of no great significance, for symbols are never sharply delineated.

Flower pollen – the favourite allergen of all hay fever sufferers – stands for the same area of experience. Flower pollen is a symbol of fertility and reproduction, just as the burgeoning springtime is the season when hay fever sufferers generally undergo their particular 'passion'. Allergens such as animal fur and pollen reveal to us that the themes of love, sexuality, instinct and fertility are hedged strongly about with fear and for this reason aggressively resisted – not allowed in.

Much the same applies to the fear of dirt, uncleanness and impurity that expresses itself in an allergy to house dust. (Compare expressions such as 'dirty jokes', 'washing one's dirty linen in public', 'living a clean life' and so on.) Just as those who are allergic endeavour to avoid their allergens, so they also avoid the corresponding areas of life – a quest in which both a sympathetic medical profession and the people around them are only too keen to help. Here, too, consequently, the power-games played by those who are ill know no limits: pets are banned, nobody can smoke any more, and so on. In this tyranny over the world around them allergy sufferers find a well-disguised field of operations for unknowingly working out their repressed aggression.

The technique of 'desensitisation' would in theory be a good idea, were it not for the fact that we need to apply ourselves to the psychological, and not the physical, level if ever we are to achieve real success. Those who are allergic can find healing only when they have learnt consciously to come to grips with the areas that they have been avoiding and devaluing – when, in short, they have managed to admit them fully into their consciousness and have finally assimilated them. One renders no service to those who are allergic by supporting them in their defence-strategies. Instead, they need to come to terms with their 'enemies' and learn to love them. The fact that allergens operate purely symbolically on the sufferer, and never on the physical, chemical level, should become perfectly clear even to the inveterate materialist when it is realised that allergies always need consciousness as a condition for their appearance. Thus, there are no allergies under narcosis, and during psychosis, equally, all allergies fade away.

On the other hand, even illustrations – such as the photo of a cat or a film-representation of a steaming locomotive – can give rise to attacks in asthmatics. The allergic reaction is totally independent of the allergic substance itself.

Most allergens are simply expressions of being alive. Sexuality, love, fertility, aggression, 'dirt' – in all these spheres life presents itself in its most vital aspects. Yet it is precisely life's drive for expression that fills those who are allergic with such fear. When it comes down to it, in other words, they are actually anti-life. Their ideal is a life that is sterile, germ-free, infertile and free of all instinct and aggression – a state which scarcely deserves the name 'life' any more. And so it is hardly surprising that allergies should in so many cases become aggravated into life-threatening forms of auto-aggression in which the bodies of such very gentle people put up so frantic a fight, and for so long, that in the end they themselves go under. At which point the self-defence, the self-isolation and self-encapsulation reach their highest point and find their culmination in the coffin – a truly allergen-free 'capsule' if ever there was one.

ALLERGY = AGGRESSION MADE FLESH

Allergy sufferers need to ask themselves the following questions:

1. Why am I refusing to tolerate aggression in my consciousness, but instead forcing it to work itself out in my body?
2. What are the areas of my life that I am so afraid of as to be avoiding them?
3. What themes are my allergens pointing to – sexuality? instinct? aggression? reproduction? 'dirt' (in the sense of the dark side of life)?
4. To what extent am I using my allergy to manipulate those around me?
5. What has become of my love and my capacity for letting in what is 'out there'?

Three

Respiration

Breathing is a rhythmic activity. It comprises two phases – inspiration and expiration. The breath is a good example of the law of polarity: the constantly alternating poles of inspiration and expiration go to make up a rhythm. In the process each pole predicates its opposite, for breathing in predicates breathing out, and vice versa. We could also say that each pole owes its life to the existence of its opposite, for if we do away with the one phase, the other disappears too. Each pole compensates for the other, and both together go to make up a whole. Breathing is rhythm, and rhythm is the basis of all living things. We could also describe the two poles of respiration in terms of *tension* and *relaxation*. The relationship between breathing in and tension on the one hand, and breathing out and relaxation on the other, becomes clear when we sigh. There is an 'inbreath-sigh' that leads to tension, and an 'outbreath-sigh' that leads to relaxation.

Seen from the point of view of the body, breathing is essentially an exchange-process: on the inbreath the oxygen in the air is brought into contact with the red blood-corpuscles, and on the outbreath carbon dioxide is released. Breathing embraces the polarity of acquisition and release, of taking and giving. And with this we have immediately discovered the most important symbolism of respiration. As Goethe put it:

> In breathing there are two blessings
> drawing breath, releasing it again,
> the one pressurises us, the other refreshes us,
> so wonderfully mixed is life.

All the ancient languages use the same word for breath as for soul or spirit. In Latin *spirare* means 'to breathe' and *spiritus* 'spirit'. We find the root of both words once again in the word 'inspiration', which literally means 'in-breathing' and so is indissolubly bound up both with breathing in and with taking in. In Greek, *psyche* means both 'breath' and 'soul'. In Sanskrit we find the word *atman*, in which we can easily detect the link with the German word *atmen* (to breathe). In Hindi a person who has attained perfection is called a *mahatma*, which literally means both 'great soul' and 'great breath'. Also from the ancient Indian teachings we learn that the breath is the bearer of our personal life-force, which the Indians call *prana*. In the biblical creation account we are told that God breathed his divine breath into the clod of earth that he had formed and in so doing made Adam a 'living soul'.

This image shows very clearly how the physical body, the formal aspect, has something *breathed into it* that does not derive from the material universe – the divine breath. It is only this 'breath', issuing from beyond the created world, that turns us into living, animated beings. And here we are very close to the secret of respiration. The breath is neither part of us, nor does it belong to us. It is not the breath that is in us, but *we who are in the breath*. Through the breath we are constantly linked to something that lies beyond the created world, beyond all form. It is the breath that sees to it that this link with the metaphysical world (literally, with that which lies *beyond nature*) is not severed. We live in the breath as in a mighty womb that extends far beyond our tiny, limited existence, for it is that life, that last great secret, that we can neither explain nor define, but only experience by opening ourselves to it and allowing it to flood through us. The breath is the umbilical cord through which this life flows into us. It is the breath that ensures that we remain true to that relationship.

That is where its true significance lies. The breath preserves us from totally cutting ourselves off, from shutting ourselves in to the point of making the frontiers of our *I* totally impenetrable. However keen we are constantly to box ourselves into our ego, the breath forces us to maintain our link with the *not-I*. We need to be conscious of the fact that we are breathing in the very same air that our enemies are breathing out. It is the self-same air, too, that the animals and plants are breathing. The breath continually connects us to everything else. However much we should like to mark out personal limits for ourselves, the breath links us with each and everything. Whether we like it or not, the air we breathe binds us all together. And so the breath also has something to do with *contact* and *relationship*.

This contact between what comes from 'out there' and our own bodies takes place in the lung-vesicles (the alveoli). Our lungs have an internal surface area of some seventy square metres, whereas the surface of our skin measures only one and a half to two square metres. The lungs are thus our largest organ of contact.

If we look at them more closely we can also see the fine distinctions between these two human contact organs, the lungs and the skin. Skin contact is a much more direct and restricted form of contact. It is more formal and intensive than that of the lungs – and at the same time subject to our will. We have the choice of touching other people or of leaving them alone. On the other hand the contact that we establish through the lungs is more indirect, yet mandatory for all that. We cannot prevent it, even if the other person seems so awful as to 'take our breath away'. In fact disease-symptoms often get shunted to and fro between the two contact organs of lungs and skin. A skin eruption that is suppressed can show up as asthma and then, once treated, change back into a skin eruption again. Like skin eruptions, asthma is an expression of the self-same problem – contact, touch, relationship. The reluctance to make contact via breathing may well show up in such forms as spasm during the outbreath, as happens in the case of asthma.

If we go on to listen more closely to those figures of speech that have to do with breathing or air, we find that there are situations in which we 'can't get our breath' or 'can no longer breathe freely'. And at this point we begin to touch on the theme of freedom and restriction. With our first breath we start life: with our last breath we end it. But with our first breath we also take our first step into the outside world, freeing ourselves from our symbiotic union with our mother: we become independent, self-sufficient, free. Any difficulty in drawing breath is often a sign of fear – fear of taking a first personal step towards freedom and independence. In such cases freedom has the effect of 'taking our breath away' – that is, of engendering fear through its sheer unfamiliarity. The same link between freedom and breath can be seen in those who emerge from some kind of restriction into a space that gives them a feeling of freedom – or indeed into the freedom of the fresh air: the first thing they do is take a deep breath, for at last they can 'breathe freely' again.

Even the expression 'Give me air!', which often comes to us in constricted circumstances, expresses a hunger for freedom and room to move.

If we are to sum up, then, the main themes that respiration symbolises are:

> Rhythm in the sense of 'both/and'
> Tension – relaxation
> Taking – giving

Contact – resistance
Freedom – constriction

RESPIRATION – ASSIMILATION OF LIFE

In the event of breath-related illness, ask yourself the following questions:

1. What is it that takes my breath away?
2. What is it that I am unwilling to accept?
3. What is it that I am unwilling to give out?
4. What is it that I am unwilling to come into contact with?
5. Am I afraid to take a step towards some new freedom?

Bronchial Asthma

Following these general observations on respiration we now propose to turn our attention in more detail to the specific symptomatology of bronchial asthma – an illness which has always provided a particularly striking example of a psycho-somatic relationship. In Braütigam's words:

> The term *bronchial asthma* refers to a kind of suffocation-fit characterised by wheezing during expiration. It is predicated by a constriction of the small bronchi and bronchioles, which can be caused by a cramping of the smooth musculature, an inflammatory itching of the airways and an allergic swelling and secretion on the part of the mucous membranes.

Patients experience asthma as a life-threatening suffocation: sufferers fight for air and breathe in gasps, with the outbreath especially throttled. In asthmatics various problem areas impinge on one another which despite their close interrelationships we propose to deal with separately for purely explanatory reasons.

1. Giving and taking

Asthmatics are trying to take too much. They breathe in so deeply that they over-inflate the lungs, so producing a cramp during the outbreath. In other words they keep taking as much as they possibly can until they are absolutely brim-full – but when it comes to having to giving it all back again they clam up.

117

We can clearly see here how the balance is disturbed: the polarities of giving and taking have to correspond if ever they are to form a rhythm. The law of change depends on inner balance, and every imbalance interrupts the flow. In asthmatics the flow of breath is interrupted by the very fact that they are too concerned with taking, and consequently overdo it. They can then no longer give back what they have taken and consequently are also unable to take any more of what they are so keen to have. During the inbreath we take in oxygen; during the outbreath we give out carbon dioxide. Those who are asthmatic are trying to hang on to everything and thereby poisoning themselves through their inability to give back out what they have used. This taking without giving leads literally to a feeling of suffocation.

There are many for whom the disproportion between giving and taking which is so vividly embodied in asthma is a theme that could well pay thinking about. It seems so simple, and yet this is where so many of us come to grief. No matter what it is that we are determined to have – be it money, fame, knowledge, wisdom – the giving and the taking have to be in balance if what we have taken is not to suffocate us. We receive only in the same measure as we give. The moment the giving stops and the flow is interrupted, the inflow stops as well. How pitiable are those who are determined to take everything they know with them to the grave! They guard so anxiously what little they have managed to scratch together, while denying themselves the abundance that awaits all those who have learnt to give back what they have received in transmuted form. If only we could all realise that there is more than enough of everything for everybody!

If we lack anything, then it is only because we have cut ourselves off from it. Take asthmatics as a case in point. What are they fighting for? Air – even though there is so much of it about. And yet there are many of us who still persist in holding our breath for more . . .

2. The attempt to shut oneself off

Asthma can be experimentally induced in anybody at all simply by giving them irritating gases such as ammonia to breathe. Once a given concentration has been reached there is a universal reflex defence-reaction consisting of a combination of diaphragm paralysis, bronchial constriction and mucus secretion. This is known as the Kretschmer reflex. This reflex amounts to a closing down and a shutting down so as not to let in something from outside. In the case of ammonia this is a sensible, life-preserving reaction, but in asthmatics it occurs at a very much lower threshold-level. As a result they unconsciously treat even the most harmless substances in the world around them as life-threatening and immediately shut themselves off from them. We have already dealt in some detail with the meaning of allergy in the last chapter, and so it suffices here to recall once again the general theme of resistance and fear. For it is indeed the case that asthma is, in general, very close to being an allergy.

In Greek, asthma is referred to as 'tight-chestedness': in Latin the word for 'tight' is *angustus*, to which the word 'anxiety' is closely related. Moreover, the Latin *angustus* is also to be found in the terms *angina* (tonsillitis) and *angina pectoris* (a painful heart condition caused by constriction of the coronary arteries). In German, meanwhile, the words *Angst* (fear, anxiety) and *eng* (tight, narrow) are inseparably linked. Thus, the tightness that is characteristic of asthma also has a great deal to do with fear – fear of letting in particular aspects of life, much as in the case of the various allergens already mentioned above. Asthmatics take the process of shutting themselves off ever further and further until it eventually reaches its climax in death. Death represents their ultimate opportunity to shut themselves off, to insulate themselves from the world of the living. (In this connection it may be of some interest to note that people suffering from relatively mild asthma can get very annoyed when told that their asthma is not life-threatening and that there is little chance of their dying from it for they attach great value to the life-threatening nature of their illness!)

3. Lust for power and feelings of smallness

Asthmatics have a strong domineering streak which they nevertheless refuse to admit to, and which is consequently forced down into the body, where it in due course reappears as the asthmatic's typical 'over-inflation'. This over-inflation reveals quite graphically the arrogance and the lust for power which they have been so careful to expunge from their consciousness. It is for this reason that they so often take refuge in idealism and formalism. The moment asthmatics are faced with another person's lust for power and dominance, however (Like for like!), the shock goes to their lungs and robs them of speech – that self-same speech which is modulated by the outbreath. They can no longer manage to breathe out – it literally takes their breath away.

Asthmatics use the symptoms of their illness to exert power over the world around them. Pets have to be got rid of, every speck of dust has to be removed, nobody is allowed to smoke, and so on.

This power-drive eventually comes to a head in life-threatening attacks which occur at just those moments when asthmatics are confronted with their own lust for power. These blackmail attacks (for that is what they are) are highly dangerous to patients themselves, in that they place them in life-threatening situations which they are often unable to bring back under control again. It is always striking how far those who are ill are prepared to damage themselves in order to exercise power. In psychotherapy an attack is often the last resort when those concerned are getting too close to the truth.

Meanwhile this close connection between the exercise of power and self-sacrifice reveals to us something of the ambivalence of such an unconscious domineering streak. For alongside the development of the power-drive and the urge constantly to inflate and puff oneself up more and more, the opposite tendency – namely a sense of impotence, smallness and helplessness – also grows in exactly the same proportion. Consciously to realise and to accept that feeling of smallness is thus one of the lessons that asthmatics need to learn.

After the illness has persisted for quite a long time, a broadening and consolidation of the thorax can ensue – generally referred to as 'barrel-chestedness'. Solid and powerful though the resultant impression may be, the lack of elasticity involved actually permits only very limited amounts of air to be breathed in and out. The conflict between pretension and reality could hardly be embodied in more graphic form.

Beneath this puffing of oneself up there is also a goodly ration of aggression. People who are asthmatic have never learnt to articulate their aggressive impulses adequately on the linguistic level. Consequently not only are they anxious to 'give themselves airs'; they feel 'fit to burst'. Yet every move to give adequate expression to their aggression by yelling or complaining 'sticks in their throat'. And so these aggressive forms of self-expression regress to the level of the body, where they emerge into the light of day in the form of coughing and expectoration. Here we need only reflect on such idioms as 'to be speechless with rage', to 'give somebody a blasting' or to 'spit in somebody's face'.

In addition, aggression shows up in the allergic component that also often goes with asthma.

4. Resistance to the dark areas of life

Asthmatics love everything that is pure, clean, bright and sterile, and tend to avoid everything that is deep, dark or earthy – an attitude that is generally reflected in their choice of allergens. They would dearly love to spend their entire lives in regions so exalted as to make it unnecessary ever again to come into contact with the lower pole of existence. By and large, therefore, they are head-orientated people (the doctrine of the elements assigns thinking to the element 'air'). Sexuality, which is just as clearly the province of the lower pole, is displaced upwards by asthmatics into the chest, as a result of which extra mucus is excreted at this level. Patients then expel this overly 'high-level' mucus via the mouth. The originality of this solution immediately becomes apparent to anybody who has come to appreciate the correspondence between the mouth and the genitals (a topic with which we shall be dealing in more detail in a later chapter).

Asthmatics long for clean air. They would much prefer to live up in the mountains (a wish that is often fulfilled under the name of 'climatic therapy'). Here their domineering streak feels at home, too, as they stand on the summit looking down on all the dark goings-on deep in the valley below – up here where they are at a safe distance from it all, where the air is still pure, far removed from the abyss where instinct and sexuality reign, high in the mountains where life reduces itself to sheer, uncomplicated minerality. This is where asthmatics live out for real the 'high-flight' that they have always striven for, latterly with the scientific connivance of eager climatologists. Another of their favourite health-resorts is the seaside with its salty air. And here again we come across the same symbolism – salt, the symbol of wilderness, of minerality, of lifelessness. This is the region that asthmatics are so keen to attain – for it is life itself that makes them afraid.

Asthmatics are people who are longing for love: it is because they want to be loved that they do so much breathing in. Yet they cannot give love to others – and so they are prevented from breathing out.

What help is there then? As with all symptoms, there is but one prescription – awareness and merciless honesty towards ourselves! Once we have finally admitted to our fears, we have to stop avoiding those areas that make us afraid, and instead start facing them fairly and squarely, until we reach the point of being able to love and to integrate them. This essential process is symbolised by one naturopathic therapy that has been success-fully used in the treatment of asthma and allergies, though it is admittedly unknown to orthodox medicine – namely auto-urinary therapy. This consists of injecting patients' own urine directly into their muscles. Looked at from the symbolic view-point, it can be seen how this therapy forces patients to take back on board what they have rejected – namely their own dirt and filth – and to get to grips with it and integrate it all over again. That, certainly, can only be healthy!

ASTHMA

Questions for asthmatics to answer:
1. In which areas am I trying to take without giving?
2. Can I admit consciously to my aggressive impulses? What opportunities do I have for expressing them?
3. How am I coping with my inner conflict between domi-nance and 'smallness'?
4. Which areas of my life am I devaluing and resisting? Can I detect something of the fear that lurks behind my system of personal values?
5. Which areas of life am I trying to avoid, and which of them do I regard as filthy, ignoble and beneath me?

(Remember – whenever tightness is detectable it is actually fear. The only way to fight fear is to expand. Expansion happens when you let in what you have hitherto been avoiding!)

Colds and Influenzal Conditions

Before leaving the breathing, we propose briefly to consider the symptomatology of colds and chills, since these affect the respiratory organs most severely. Influenza and colds alike are acute inflammatory processes, and so we can tell that they are expressions of coming to grips with conflict. Consequently for the purposes of our interpretation it only remains for us at this point to consider the sites and areas where the inflammatory process occurs. Colds always arise at times of crisis when things are 'getting up our nose' or when we are feeling stuffy about something. Possibly there are some who will find the term 'times of crisis' somewhat overblown. We are of course referring here not to the more drastic life-crises, which express themselves via correspondingly major symptoms. By 'times of crisis' we simply mean those frequent, unsensational, yet – for the psyche – still important everyday situations that overstress us, and which for that reason we seek some legitimate reason to draw back from a little because they are demanding too much of us. It is because we are not prepared at the time to take up the challenge of these 'minor' everyday situations and consciously to admit to our desire to escape them that somatisation ensues: our body proceeds to live out for real our 'stuffiness' and the fact that things are 'getting up our nose'. Yet even via this route we have, however unconsciously, achieved our aim – and with the additional advantage that everybody shows great understanding of our situation, which is not something that we could necessarily have counted on had we got to work on the relevant conflict at the conscious level. For once, our cold permits us to withdraw somewhat from the particular situation that is oppressing us and to devote all our attention to ourselves. Now we can give full vent to our sensitivity on the bodily level.

And so we get a headache (under the circumstances, after all, nobody can expect us to take on yet another conscious confrontation!), our eyes start watering, everything is sore and irritated. In the end this general sensitivity can build up into so-called 'prickly catarrh'. Nobody is allowed to come too near us, nothing and nobody must touch us. The nose is blocked and makes all communication impossible (breathing itself, after all, is a form of contact!). With the threat, 'Don't come too near me, I've got a cold!' we successfully keep everybody at bay. We can give further impressive backing to this defensive attitude by sneezing, for in this way our expiration is turned into a highly aggressive defence-weapon. Even language's role as a means of communication is reduced to a minimum by the sore throat – and in any case it is useless for any further confrontation. A 'barking cough' shows clearly by its threatening tone that the joy of conversation is in our case limited at best to 'biting other people's heads off'.

With all this resistance going on, the fact that the tonsils – one of the body's most important defensive organs – are also working at top pressure is hardly surprising. In the process they swell up so much that we 'can't swallow it all any more' – a state of affairs that ought to encourage us to ask ourselves critically what it actually is that we are no longer prepared to swallow. Swallowing, after all, is an act of taking on board, of acceptance. But that is precisely what we are not prepared to do any more.*

*We are 'fed up to the back teeth with it all', we say. – tr.

Colds and chills tell us as much on every level. The aching limbs and the run-down feeling characteristic of influenza restrict all movement and often even convey via aches in the shoulders a clear impression of the weight of the problems that are being heaped on our backs and that we are no longer prepared to 'shoulder'.

In the form of pus and mucus, then, we try to rid ourselves of a whole host of problems, and the freer we become of them the more relieved we feel. The stringy mucus that originally blocked everything up and thus interrupted the flow of communication has to dissolve and become liquefied before the flow can be restored and everything be set in motion once more. So it is that every cold finishes up by setting something in train again, and signals a minor step in our development. Naturopathy is thus right to see in colds an entirely healthy cleansing process through which toxins are flushed out of the body. For on the psychological level the toxins correspond to problems which have similarly to be dissolved and expelled. Body and soul emerge from the crisis strengthened – until the next time things get up our nose, too much, that is . . .

_____ *Four* _____

Digestion

What happens in digestion is very similar to what happens in respiration. Through our breathing we take in part of the world around us, assimilate what we can of it and return what we cannot. The same thing occurs in digestion, though the digestion process is more deeply concerned with the body's physicality. The breath is ruled by the element Air, whereas the digestion belongs to the element Earth and is thus more materially orientated. By contrast with the breathing, the digestion lacks any clear rhythm. With the more sluggish Earth element the rhythmic assimilation and excretion of nutrients loses its clarity and definition.

Equally, the digestion has similarities with what the brain does, for it is the brain (or consciousness) that consumes and digests the non-material impress of the world (man does not live by bread alone!). Via the digestion, on the other hand, we deal with the world's *material* impress. Thus, digestion involves:

1. the intake of the external world's material impress
2. the discrimination of what is 'beneficial' from what is 'unbeneficial'
3. the assimilation of beneficial materials
4. the excretion of unbeneficial materials.

Before we get to closer grips with the problems that can arise in the sphere of digestion it will be useful to cast a brief glance at what food symbolises. We can learn a good deal straight away from the particular foods and dishes that people prefer or dislike (tell me what you eat and I'll tell you who you are!). It is, after all, sound practice to sharpen our vision and awareness to the point where, even in the most ordinary, everyday goings-on, we can spot the ulterior connections that link phenomena behind the scenes – for they are never accidental. If we have an appetite for something special, that fact is an expression of a quite specific affinity and is thus a statement about ourselves. If something is 'not to our taste', this antipathy is just as amenable to interpretation as any decision we may make in the course of a psychological test. Hunger is a symbol of a desire to have, to take in, an expression of a certain craving. Eating is the satisfaction of our wants through integration – through ingestion and eventual satiation.

If a person is hungry for love without having that hunger adequately requited, it reappears in the body as a hunger for sweet things. A craving for sweet things and for nibbling at dainties is always an expression of an unsatisfied hunger for love. The double meaning that attaches to the word 'sweet' and the idea of nibbling becomes particularly obvious when one considers the case of a man in love 'nibbling the ear' of his 'sweet young thing'. Love and sweetness go closely together. In children, too, a constant urge to nibble away at sweet things is a clear indication that they feel insufficiently loved. In the face of this suggestion, parents are quick to protest that 'they are doing all they can for their child'. Yet 'doing all one can' and 'loving' are not necessarily the same. Those who are always nibbling are in fact longing for love and support. This rule can safely be regarded as more reliable than any personal evaluation we might make of just how loving we are. There are even parents who over-indulge their children with sweet things and thereby announce that they are not prepared to love their child, but for this reason are ready instead to compensate him or her on another level.

People who do a lot of thinking and are engaged in intellectual work tend to have a yen for salty food and hearty eating. Those with a strongly conservative orientation prefer preserved and tinned foods, and especially smoked foods, and like strong tea (which they tend to drink unsweetened) along with tannin-rich food in general. People who prefer highly spiced and even hot foods are revealing that they are constantly on the lookout for new thrills and impressions. There are people, indeed, who are so keen on such challenges that they do not mind if they are sometimes difficult to take and 'hard to digest'. Quite the contrary is the case, however, with people who will only eat mild foods – no salt, no spices. These are people who are loth to *season* their lives with new impressions and so are determined to avoid that variety – that constant contact with new things – which is the proverbial 'spice of life'. Thus, they are anxious to avoid all challenges, and go in fear of any confrontation. This fear can escalate to the point where they adopt the purely liquid diet so characteristic of those with stomach ailments, whose personalities we shall be discussing in greater detail shortly. A liquid diet is basically baby-food – a fact which indicates clearly that the stomach sufferer has regressed to the undifferentiatedness of childhood, when there was no obligation either to be able to *de-cide* ('cut apart') or to 'get one's teeth into' anything, and one could consequently get along without chewing up food (How aggressive!) or digesting it. Such people, in other words, find adult life 'too much to stomach' – altogether 'too hard a nut to crack'.

A particular fear of fish-bones symbolises fear of aggression. A fear of pips indicates that one is afraid of problems – one is unwilling to 'get to the heart of things'. But then there is the opposite group, too – the macrobiotic brigade. These are people who are actually on the lookout for problems. They are determined to get to the heart of the matter at all costs, and so are quite amenable to solid foods. This tendency can be taken so far that an actual rejection of the problem-free areas of life can be detected: to accompany sweet desserts they demand something solid to get their teeth into. In the process, macrobiotic enthusiasts reveal a certain fear of love and tenderness, and/or a difficulty in accepting love. Meanwhile some people even manage to push their dislike of conflict to such an extreme point that they finish up by being fed intravenously in intensive care – which is undoubtedly the surest way of remaining aloof from all conflicts and becoming a mere vegetable!

The Teeth

The food first enters the mouth, where it is reduced to small pieces by the teeth. It is with the teeth that we do all our biting and chewing. Biting is a highly aggressive business, an expression of our ability to look after ourselves, get to grips with things and 'get our teeth into things'. Just as dogs bare their teeth, so we also speak of 'showing our teeth' when we reveal our willingness to stand up and fight. Bad or decaying teeth are an indication of difficulty in expressing our aggression.

This link is by no means invalidated by the point that nowadays many people have bad teeth – as can even be observed in small children. This is certainly true, yet collective symptoms merely reflect collective problems. Aggression has become a central problem in all the socially highly developed cultures of our day. There is a demand for 'social acceptability' – which in plain words means 'Repress your aggression.' When those dear fellow citizens of ours who are so peaceable and socially well-adapted repress all their aggressive urges, these re-emerge into the light of day as 'illnesses' and thus go on to affect the community at large in their new, perverted form just as much as they would have done in their original one. Consequently our clinics and hospitals are present-day society's battlefields. It is here that the repressed aggressive urges mercilessly wage war against those who harbour them. It is here that people suffer from their own malignancies – malignancies that they have spent their whole lives not daring to uncover or to deal with consciously.

No wonder, then, that we come across aggression and sexuality again and again in the vast majority of clinical profiles. It is these two problem areas that people of today most rigorously repress. It may of course be objected that both today's rising criminality and violence and also the new 'sexual wave' argue against our thesis. By way of response, however, it needs to be pointed out that not only a lack of aggression, but also its actual eruption are symptoms of its having been repressed. The two are merely different phases of the same process. Only where aggression does not need to be repressed because those concerned have from the start been allowed space to gain experience of the energies involved is it possible for them to integrate the aggressive aspects of their personalities. Aggression that has been successfully integrated then stands at the disposal of the whole personality as a source of energy and vitality, without leading either to sugary meekness at one extreme or to wild aggressive outbreaks at the other. But such a state of affairs has to be worked for, and this requires opportunities for learning and maturing through actual experience. Repressing aggression merely leads to a growth in the shadow, which we then have to come to terms with in perverted form as illness. Indeed, what we have just said applies equally to sexuality, just as it does to all the other human psychological functions.

However, let us return to the teeth, which both in the animal and in the human body represent aggression and assertiveness ('getting one's teeth into things'). Reference is often made to primitive peoples whose healthy teeth are attributed to their natural diet. But then among such peoples we also find a quite different way of coping with aggression. Even with this collective symptomatology, moreover, the state of the teeth still lends itself to individual interpretation. In addition to the aggression to which we have just been referring, the teeth also reveal to us the state of our vitality or life-force (aggression and vitality are merely two disparate aspects of one and the same force, yet the two concepts awaken quite different associations in us). Consider, for example, the expression 'Never look a gift horse in the mouth.' At the basis of this saying lies the custom of looking into a horse's mouth at the time of purchase in order to assess its age *and vitality* from the condition of its teeth. Psychoanalytical dream-interpretation similarly construes the falling out of teeth in dreams as a sign of loss of energy and potency.

Some people regularly grind their teeth at night, sometimes so vehemently that they have to be fitted with an artificial brace to stop them wearing their teeth right down. The symbolism is obvious. In our symbolic usage, 'grinding our teeth' is a well-established term for impotent aggression. Those of us who are unable to fulfil our wish to snap at people during the day are forced to grind our teeth at night to the point of wearing down and blunting those teeth that are so sharp and deadly.

Those who have bad teeth lack vitality and also the ability to 'get to grips with things' and to 'get their teeth into things'. Thus, they often find problems 'hard to chew' or 'a hard nut to crack'. Hence the German toothpaste advertisements which describe the desired end in the words 'so that you can get your teeth into things again!'

Wearing false teeth, meanwhile, makes it possible for us to simulate a vitality and a self-assertiveness that we no longer possess. Yet this act – like all such prostheses – remains a deception, and is rather like the well-known trick of proclaiming the fierceness of one's timid but beloved lapdog by fixing a notice saying 'Beware of the dog' to the garden gate. Buying false teeth is merely paying somebody else to 'show your teeth' for you.

The gums provide the foundation in which the teeth are embedded. By the same token, then, the gums represent the necessary basis for our vitality and aggression, for our native confidence and self-assurance. So long as we lack our full measure of native confidence and self-assurance we shall never succeed in getting actively to grips with the core of our problems, or have the courage to 'crack hard nuts' or 'stand up and fight'. It is confidence that has to provide the necessary basis for this ability, just as the gums provide the basis for the teeth. But this the gums cannot do if they themselves are so sensitive and delicate that they bleed at the slightest provocation. Blood is the symbol of life itself, and so bleeding gums make it perfectly obvious that our innate confidence and self-assurance are liable to drain away as soon as the slightest demands are placed on our vitality.

Swallowing

Once the food has been chewed up by the teeth and mixed with saliva we swallow down the resultant pulp. Swallowing is a form of integration, of ingestion: to swallow, in other words, is to incorporate. All the while we retain something in our mouths we can spit it out again. But once we have swallowed it down it is no easy matter to reverse the process. Big pieces, meanwhile, we find 'hard to swallow'. Indeed, if something is too big we 'just can't swallow it any more'. There are many occasions in life when we have to swallow things that we would rather not – unwelcome pieces of information, for example. There is plenty of bad news that makes us 'swallow hard'.

In just such cases swallowing whatever is involved comes easier for the accompaniment of a little liquor – and all the more so if it amounts to a 'good swig'. We often say of people who drink a lot that they are 'guzzlers' who simply 'gulp it down'. The swigging of alcoholics is for the most part designed to make it easier to swallow some other matter that is hard to swallow, or even to supplant the need to swallow it at all. We drink liquor because there is something else in our lives that we cannot and will not swallow. In this way alcoholics replace eating with drinking (heavy drinking leads to loss of appetite). In place of swallowing solid food they substitute the much gentler, easier form of swallowing that is offered them by the bottle.

There are a whole range of conditions affecting our ability to swallow – as, for example, a 'lump in the throat' or sore throats of the angina type, all of which give the feeling that we 'can't swallow it any more'. In such cases sufferers would always do well to ask themselves, 'What is it in my life that I am currently unable or unwilling to swallow?' Among other swallowing problems, incidentally, there is one particularly original variant which comes in the form of gulping air, known technically as 'aerophagy' (literally 'air-eating'). The term itself shows quite clearly what is involved. Those concerned are not prepared to swallow or assimilate something, but still feign a willingness to do so by 'swallowing air'. This hushed-up resistance to swallowing whatever it is then goes on to express itself somewhat later in the form of belching and anal venting (in other words we 'create a stink').

Nausea and Vomiting

Once we have swallowed the food and ingested it, it can nevertheless turn out to be 'hard to digest' and to 'lie like a stone in our stomach'. But then a stone – like a pip – is a symbol for a problem (the proverbial 'stumbling-block'). We all know how a problem can 'churn up our guts' and ruin our appetite. Our appetite is highly dependent on psychological circumstances. There are many idioms that reflect this analogy between what goes on at the psychological and somatic levels: 'I've no appetite for it,' for example, or 'Just thinking about it makes me sick,' or even 'I'm sick of the sight of him.' Nausea signals the rejection of something that we do not want and that consequently 'lies uneasy in the stomach'. Wild, indiscriminate gastronomic self-indulgence can lead to nausea too. Nor does this apply on the physical level only: we can just as easily stuff our minds with too much unsuitable material at once, to the point where it all starts 'disagreeing with us' because we 'cannot digest it'.

Nausea reaches its culmination in the vomiting of food. In the process we get rid of all those things and impressions that we do not want and are unready to incorporate or integrate. Vomiting is an overwhelming expression of resistance and refusal. As the Jewish painter Max Liebermann put it in connection with political and artistic conditions following 1933, 'I want to spew up more than I can possibly eat!'

Vomiting is a refusal to accept. This link is also quite plain in the case of the well-known 'morning-sickness' that is associated with pregnancy. It represents the expression of a degree of unconscious resistance towards the developing child – or indeed towards the male sperm that one perhaps did not completely want to 'incorporate' in the first place. Pursuing this line of thought further, morning-sickness could also be seen as expressing a woman's rejection of her own female role – of motherhood itself.

The Stomach

Assuming that we have not vomited it up again, the next place that our food reaches is the stomach, whose primary function is reception. It takes in all the impressions that come from outside and receives whatever is to be digested. The ability to receive requires openness, passivity and willingness (in the sense of self-surrender). With these properties the stomach represents the feminine role. Just as the masculine principle is character-ised by activity and the ability to radiate energy (the element Fire), so the feminine principle expresses receptivity, self-surrender, susceptibility and the ability to receive and contain (the element Water). On the psychological level it is the ability to feel and the world of feelings generally (NB *not* the emotions!) that embodies the feminine element in this connection. If we drive out of our consciousness the capacity to feel, this function descends to the bodily level, where it is the stomach that now has to take in and digest not merely the impress of our physical food, but our psychological feelings too. In such cases it is not just that 'the way to a man's heart is through his stomach': we have 'gut feelings' too, and get 'eaten up inside', so leading eventually to the phenomenon of the 'worry-guts'.

Alongside its capacity for reception, we also find in the stomach a further function that demands to be assigned to the masculine pole – namely the production and release of stomach-acid. Acid attacks, corrodes (literally 'gnaws away'), stings, disintegrates – it is unequivocally aggressive. When nothing suits us and things are going very much against the grain we become 'sour inside'. If we fail to deal consciously with this sense of annoyance or to transform it into out-and-out aggression, we have to 'swallow our anger', in which case our aggression and sourness become embodied in stomach acid. The stomach undergoes an acid reaction, producing attacking juices on the physical level in an attempt to digest and deal with purely non-material feelings – a difficult undertaking that causes a great deal of belching and upward pressure by way of reminding us that feelings are better not swallowed at all, and that the stomach is best left to get on with its business of real digestion. The acid comes up again, in other words, simply because it needs to be ex-pressed.

Yet this is where people with stomach ailments have problems. They lack the capacity to cope consciously with what is annoying them or with their own aggressive urges, and thus are unable to resolve their conflicts and problems on their own account. Such people either do not express their aggression at all (they 'get eaten up inside') or they show exaggerated aggression: yet neither extreme is of much help to them in bringing their problems to a proper resolution, since they lack any foundation of self-confidence and security for coming to personal grips with their conflicts – a problem which we have already discussed in connection with the teeth and gums. Everybody knows that badly chewed food is difficult for an irritated and over-acid stomach to take. But to chew is to be aggressive. If, consequently, there is a lack of this aggressive chewing-behaviour, the task of expressing the aggression falls to the stomach, which duly goes on to produce extra acid.

Stomach sufferers are people who are unwilling to enter

into conflicts. They are unconsciously pining for the conflict-free world of childhood. Their stomachs crave liquid food once again. And so such sufferers live on strained foods – on food that has already demonstrated how innocuous it is by passing through a sieve or filter. Thus, there can be no more 'hard nuts' left in it to crack. The problems have all been left behind in the sieve. Stomach sufferers will tolerate no raw food – it is much too coarse, too basic, too dangerous. All food must first be cooked to death – aggressively pre-treated – before they will venture anywhere near it. Even wholemeal bread is too hard to digest: it still involves too many problems. All hot and spicy foods, alcohol, coffee, nicotine and sweet things generally are far too irritating for stomach sufferers to face. Living and eating have alike to be free of all challenges. Stomach acidity leads to a feeling of pressure that prevents the intake of any further *impress-ions*.

The taking of antacid medicines generally leads to belching, which duly brings relief. Belching, after all, is a form of aggressive self-expression vis-à-vis the outside world. It is a way of 'giving oneself air' and reducing the internal pressure. The tranquilliser therapy so often applied by academic medicine (Valium, for example) likewise demonstrates the same relationship. The effect of the medicine is to break the link between the psyche and the biochemical realm (so-called *psycho-vegetative decoupling*) – a step that in severe cases is also undertaken by surgical means, with operations being performed on people with ulcers to sever the particular nerve-stems responsible for acid-production (vagotomy). In the case of both forms of conventional medical intervention the link between feeling and the stomach is broken, so that the stomach no longer has to digest the patient's feelings in physical form. The stomach is protected from external stimuli. This close connection between psyche and stomach secretions has been well enough known ever since Pavlov's experiments. (By synchronising feeding with the sound of a bell Pavlov was able to induce so-called conditioned reflexes in the dogs that were his research-subjects, so that after a time the bell-tone alone was enough to produce the stomach-secretions which the sight of food normally elicited.)

The basic tendency to direct our feelings and aggressions not outwards, but inwards against ourselves, eventually leads to the growth of gastric ulcers (though these are not in fact growths, or tumours, but penetrations of the stomach-wall). In gastric ulcers what is digested is not matter from outside, but the stomach-wall itself – we are *digesting ourselves*, in other words. 'Flaying ourselves alive' would in fact be a good way of describing it. What stomach sufferers need to learn is to make themselves aware of their own feelings, to get to conscious grips with their conflicts and consciously to digest incoming impressions. Furthermore, ulcer patients need not only to become aware of, but actually to admit to, their desire for infantile dependence and maternal security and their longing to be loved and cared for – even (indeed, especially) if these desires are well-hidden behind a facade of independence, competence and pride.* In this, as ever, the stomach speaks the truth.

STOMACH DISORDERS AND DIGESTIVE COMPLAINTS

If you are suffering from stomach disorders or digestive complaints, you would do well to ask yourself the following questions:

1. What is it that I am unable or unwilling to swallow?
2. Is something 'eating me up inside?'
3. How good am I at handling my feelings?
4. What I am feeling so 'sour' about?
5. How am I coping with my aggression?
6. To what extent am I deliberately avoiding conflicts?
7. Is there in me a repressed longing for the conflict-free paradise of childhood – a paradise in which I am given nothing but love and care, without ever having to 'eat my heart out'?

The Small and Large Intestines

It is in the small intestine that the actual digestion of food occurs via a process of splitting it up into its constituent parts (analysis) and of eventual assimilation. What is particularly striking here is the apparent similarity between the small intestine and the brain. Both have identical jobs and functions: the brain digests impressions on the non-physical level, while the small intestine digests all the various material inputs. Disorders in the region of the small intestine should thus raise the question of whether we are being too analytical, for it is in the nature of the small intestine's job to analyse, to split apart and to go into detail. People with disorders of the small intestine incline for the most part towards excessive analysis and criticism: they are always

'He had to swallow his pride', we say. – tr.

finding fault with things. The small intestine is also a good indicator of any fears that we may have for our own survival. It is in the small intestine, after all, that the food is made use of and 'exploited'. Yet behind too great an emphasis on exploiting and making good use of things there always stand fears for one's own survival – a fear, that is, of not being able to get enough out of things, a fear of going hungry. It is much rarer for problems with the small intestine to point to the opposite – an *under*-developed critical faculty – though this *is* the case where the 'fatty stools' of pancreatic deficiency are concerned.

One of the commonest of the symptoms associated with the small intestine is diarrhoea. In vulgar parlance we say, 'He's scared shitless', or even 'He's messing his pants'. 'Shit', in fact, corresponds to fear. In diarrhoea, then, we have a pointer to some problem connected with fear. When we are afraid, we no longer take time to analyse incoming impressions. Instead we let them all through undigested. Nothing 'hangs around' any more. We withdraw to a quiet, lonely place where we can 'let things run their course'. In the process we lose a lot of fluid – that fluid which symbolises the flexibility that is needed if we are to extend the constricting (and thus worrying) confines of the ego and so overcome our fear. We have already discussed the way in which fear is always bound up with tightness and constriction. The therapy for fear is always to let go and expand, to become flexible and let be. The therapy for diarrhoea is thus no more than to administer large quantities of fluid. In this way patients acquire that fluidity that they need in order to extend the confines within which they are currently cowering. Diarrhoea, whether chronic or acute, always tells us that we are afraid, over-anxious to hang on to things: it teaches us to let go and let things run their course.

By the time the food reaches the large intestine, the digestion as such is already finished. This is merely where the water is extracted from the food's indigestible remnants. The most widespread disorder that affects this part of the system is constipation. Ever since Freud, psychoanalysis has been interpreting defecation as an act of giving and generosity. The fact that excrement has something to do with money soon becomes clear as soon as we think of the expression 'Where there's muck there's brass', or equally of the story of the Golden Ass which allegedly excreted gold pieces instead of stools. Similarly, German folk-tradition connects accidentally treading in dog's mess with the prospect of unexpected riches, just as British folk-wisdom regards being hit by bird-droppings as a good-luck sign. These indications alone should suffice to make clear without any further theoretical justification the symbolic link between money and excreta, as equally between the act of excretion and giving things away. Constipation, consequently, is an expression of a reluctance to give things away, of a desire to hang on to things, and thus always touches on the problem area of avarice. Constipation today is a very widespread symptom from which the majority of us have suffered at some time or other. It shows that we are hanging on too tightly to material things and are unable to let go on the physical level.

There is also a further important symbolic significance to the large intestine, however. Just as the small intestine corresponds to conscious, analytical thinking, so the large intestine reflects the unconscious – literally in terms of the 'underworld'. The unconscious has always been regarded symbolically as the realm of the dead. The large intestine is similarly a 'realm of the dead', for in it are to be found all those materials that cannot be brought to life. It is also a place where fermentation can occur. Fermentation is a process both of rotting and of dying. If the large intestine is the bodily symbol for the unconscious, for our 'night side', so the faeces correspond to the contents of the unconscious. At which point we can recognise quite clearly the next meaning of constipation – the fear of letting unconscious contents see the light of day. It represents an attempt to keep unconscious, repressed contents locked up within ourselves. Psychological impressions are stored up within us, and we are no longer able to get shot of them. Sufferers from constipation are literally unable to leave their contents behind them. For this reason psychotherapy is helped considerably by first of all using physical means to free any existing constipation so that, by analogy, the contents of the unconscious can also be brought to light. Constipation shows us that we have difficulties with giving and letting go, that we are hanging on both to material things and to unconscious contents which we do not want to come to light.

Ulcerative colitis is the name of an inflammatory condition of the large intestine which starts in acute form but tends to become chronic, and is accompanied by bodily pain and by blood and slime (mucus) in the stools. Here again common parlance reveals deep psychosomatic knowledge. We all know people who are 'slimy'. They are people who are prepared to 'lick our arses' in order to ingratiate themselves with us – yet this involves them in sacrificing their own personalities and giving up all life of their own in order to live other people's lives for them. By dint of 'licking our arses' they are, in effect, living in symbiotic union with us. Blood and slime are living substances, the primal symbols of life itself. (The myths of a number of primitive peoples recount how all life originally developed out of slime.) People who are losing blood and slime are people who are afraid to *real-ise* their own lives and personalities. Living our own lives, after all, demands that we take up our own position vis-à-vis other people, which inevitably entails a certain degree of isolation (and thus a loss of symbiosis). But that is precisely what colitis patients are most afraid of. It is out of fear that they then go on to 'sweat blood' via the intestine. By way of the intestine (and the unconscious) they are sacrificing the symbols of their own life – namely blood and slime. The only thing that can help them is the realisation that we all have to accept responsibility for our own lives – or else lose them.

The Pancreas

Another organ that pertains to the digestion is the pancreas, which has two main functions. The exocrine part of it produces the vital digestive juices whose activity reveals a clearly aggressive nature. The endocrine part of the pancreas – the groups of cells known as the *islets of Langerhans* – produce insulin. It is under-production on the part of these cells that leads to the widely known symptomatology of diabetes. The word 'diabetes' comes from the Greek verb *diabeinein*, which means 'to throw through' or 'to go through'. Once upon a time this disease was also known as *glycosuria* – meaning, in effect, 'sugar run-out'. If we now recall the food symbolism already set out above, we can translate the term 'sugar run-out' as a running-out (a failure) of love. For want of insulin, diabetics cannot assimilate the sugar that they take in via their food: the sugar passes straight through them, to be excreted back out again by way of the urine. Thus, we have merely to substitute the word 'love' for 'sugar' to have the diabetic's general problem area neatly summed up. Sweet things are merely substitutes for those other 'sweet things' that help to ensure that life is 'sweet' for us. Behind the desire of diabetics to enjoy sweet things, and their simultaneous inability to assimilate sugar and absorb it into their own body-cells, stands an unsatisfied desire for love, along with an inability to accept love and absorb it unreservedly. Diabetics are typically obliged to live on 'substitute foods' – substitutes, that is, for what they really want. Diabetes leads to an over-acidification of the whole body, to the point of eventual coma. We are already acquainted with acid as a symbol for aggression. Again and again we come across this polarity between love and aggression, between sugar and acid (and thus mythologically between Venus and Mars). The body warns us that those who are without love become sour – or, to put it even more bluntly, that those who have no tolerance soon become intolerable themselves.

The only people who can accept love are people who can also give it – but those of us who are diabetic give out love only in the form of unassimilated sugar in the urine. Those who are insufficiently prepared to 'let things pass' find that the sugar lets *itself* pass – in this case through their bodies (in the form of glycosuria). Diabetics want love (in the form of sweet things), yet do not trust themselves actively to pursue it ('I really musn't have anything sweet!'). And so they long for it all the more ('I should like to so much, but I musn't!'), yet are unable to get it because they have never learnt to love themselves. And so love passes them by – they have to excrete the sugar that they have failed to assimilate. Not that this is really anything to be sour about . . .

The Liver

As an organ of enormously diverse functions, the liver is not a particularly simple one for us to consider. It is not only one of the largest organs in the human body, but the central organ of the intermediate metabolism or – to put it more graphically – the body's laboratory. Let us sketch out briefly here its more important functions:

1. *The storage of energy*: The liver produces glycogen (starch) and stores it (up to some five hundred kilocalories of it). At the same time the carbohydrates that we have absorbed are turned into fat and laid down as part of the body's various fatty deposits.

2. *The generation of energy*: The liver produces glucose (energy) from the amino acids and fatty constituents that we absorb via our food. All this fat finds its way to the liver, where it can be burnt to produce energy.

3. *Protein-processing*: The liver is able not merely to take proteins apart but also to synthesise new ones. Thus, the liver is the connecting link between the proteins of the animal and plant kingdoms on the one hand (from which our food comes) and human protein on the other. Each kind of

protein is in fact quite distinct, yet the building-blocks from which all protein is constructed – the amino acids – are universal. (By way of analogy, a whole variety of individual types of house – the proteins – can be built from the same bricks – the amino acids). The individual differences between plant, animal and human protein are a function of the various patterns in which the amino acids are arranged, with the precise sequence being encoded in the DNA.

4. *Detoxification*: Both foreign poisons and those produced by the body itself are de-activated and made soluble in the liver so that they can be excreted via the gall-bladder or the kidneys. In addition, bilirubin (a by-product of the decomposition of the red pigment haemoglobin) has to be changed in the liver into a form that can be excreted. Any interruption of this process leads to jaundice. Finally the liver synthesises urea, which is excreted via the kidneys.

So much for a potted summary of the most important functions of this many-sided organ. Let us begin our symbolic interpretation, then, with the last-mentioned point, namely detoxification. The liver's ability to undertake this process presupposes a capacity to distinguish and evaluate, for detoxification is impossible if what is poisonous and what is non-poisonous cannot be told apart. Liver disturbances and diseases therefore suggest problems of evaluation and assessment, and indicate a faulty estimation of what is useful or harmful (an inability to tell 'food' from 'poison'). Clearly, all the while we can tell what is good for us and how much of it we can process and digest, the question of 'too much' never arises. But the moment the point of excess is reached the liver invariably takes ill: too much fat, too much to eat, too much alcohol, too many drugs and so on. A sick liver shows us that we are taking in more of something than we can possibly cope with: it is an index of immoderation, exaggerated ideas of expansion and over-lofty ideals.

The liver is our distributor of energy. It is precisely this energy and life-force, consequently, that liver sufferers lose out on. They lose their sexual potency, their love of eating and drinking. They lose interest in all those areas that have to do with expressing the life within them – and in this way their symptomatology is already starting to correct their main problem, which is *excess*. It is the body's reaction to their immoderation and delusions of grandeur, duly teaching them to let go of this excess. Because the normal blood-clotting factors are no longer being produced, the blood becomes 'thin', and so their blood – their very life-blood – literally drains away. From their illness patients thus learn moderation, patience and restraint (in sex, in eating and in drinking) – a process which we can see vividly illustrated in the case of hepatitis.

In addition, the liver has a strong symbolic link with the spheres of philosophy and religion, though this conclusion may not strike too many people as very obvious at first sight. Let us though, recall the process of protein-synthesis. Protein is the basic building-block of all life. It is manufactured from the amino acids. The liver manufactures human protein out of the plant and animal protein in our food by altering the spatial arrangement of the amino acid molecules. In other words, while retaining the individual building-blocks (the amino acids) the liver alters the way in which they are put together and so brings off a qualitative leap, or evolutionary advance, from the plant and animal kingdoms to the human one. Despite this evolutionary advance, however, the building-blocks' identity is still preserved, so maintaining the link with the source. Protein-synthesis is thus a total, microcosmic illustration of what, at the macrocosmic level, we refer to as 'evolution'. Through a re-arrangement and alteration of the qualitative pattern the self-same 'original building-blocks' are used to create the whole, infinite variety of forms. Because the raw material itself remains constant, everything is always linked to everything else – and so, as ancient wisdom has it, all is in one and one in all (*pars pro toto*).

Another expression for this *real-isation* is the word *religio* – literally 'binding back together'. Religion seeks to reconnect us to the source, to the origin, to the All-One, and rediscovers this connection by virtue of the fact that the diversity which separates us from the Unity is, in the last resort, just an illusion (*maya*) – and one which comes into being thanks only to the play of the various arrangements (patterns) of the one common essence. For this reason the way back can only be discovered by those who have seen through the illusion of the world's formal diversity. The many and the One, then – it is in the field of tension between these two poles that the liver operates.

LIVER DISEASES

If you are suffering from a liver problem, ask yourself the following questions:

1. In what areas have I lost my capacity for accurate assessment and evaluation?

2.   In what respects can I no longer distinguish between what is good for me and what is 'poisonous'?

3.   Where have I been taking things to excess? To what extent am I aiming too high (delusions of grandeur!) and generally going beyond the limit?

4.   Am I having due regard to my *religio*, my connection with the source, or is the world of diversity getting in the way of my *in-sight*? Are philosophical considerations playing too small a part in my life?

5.   Am I lacking in confidence?

The Gall-Bladder

The gall-bladder collects the bile that is produced by the liver. But the bile cannot find its way into the digestive system if the bile-ducts are obstructed, as is often the case where gallstones are present. As we know from common speech, meanwhile, bile (or gall) corresponds to aggression – 'And then she had the gall to accuse me of it!', we say. Those who are 'choleric' are so called specifically after this bilious, blocked aggression.

It is notable that gallstones more often appear in women, whereas in men kidney-stones are more frequent. Moreover, the incidence of gallstones is significantly higher in married women with children than in unmarried women. These statistical observations may perhaps make the course of our interpretation somewhat easier. Energy needs to flow. If energy is prevented from flowing, an energy-blockage results. If an energy-blockage finds no outlet for some time, the energy has a tendency to solidify. Deposits and stones within the body are always manifestations of congealed energy. Gallstones are fossilised bits of aggression. ('Energy' and 'aggression' are almost identical concepts. Let us be clear, though, that words such as 'aggression' have no negative connotations here: we need aggression just as much as we need bile – or teeth, for that matter!)

The frequency of gallstones in married women with families is thus hardly surprising. To such women the family is a structure which seems to prevent them from letting their energy and their aggression flow naturally. Familiar situations turn into obligations which they do not trust themselves to shrug off again, and so all their energies congeal and fossilise. In colic, consequently, patients are forced to make up for all the things that they have never previously managed to pluck up the courage to do. By way of violent movements and loud yells the repressed energy is once more set in motion. As ever, illness makes us honest!

Anorexia Nervosa

We propose to conclude our chapter on the digestion with a classic psychosomatic illness which owes its charms to a mixture of originality and sheer danger (after all, 20 per cent of all female patients suffering from this illness still die of it!) – namely *anorexia nervosa*. In this illness the humour and irony that are inherent in every illness come to the surface particularly vividly: patients refuse to eat because they have no wish to, and die of it without ever getting the feeling that they are actually ill. It all shows a certain magnanimity. The relations and doctors of such patients generally find such magnanimity much harder to come by. For the most part their sole anxiety is to try and convince the anorexics in question of the advantages of eating and living, in the process pushing their love of their fellow human beings to the point of clinically force-feeding them. (Anyone who fails to see the humour in this must be a poor observer of the antics we get up to!)

Anorexia nervosa occurs almost exclusively in female patients. In fact it is a typically female illness. The patients involved (most of them still at puberty) are remarkable for their peculiar eating habits – or rather for their *non*-eating habits. Their refusal to accept food is motivated by a desire – part conscious, part unconscious – to stay slim.

This strict refusal to eat anything meanwhile tends to turn into its opposite: as soon as they are alone and are not being seen or observed, they start gobbling down enormous quantities of food. At night they will empty the fridge and eat absolutely everything in sight. And yet they have no wish to keep the food down, and so duly see to it that they vomit it all back up again. They think up all sorts of tricks to deceive the worried people around them about their eating-habits. It is for the most part extremely difficult to arrive at any accurate picture of what anorexics are really eating or not eating, or to establish when they are satisfying their cravings and when they are not.

When they *do* eat, though, they prefer things that hardly deserve the name of food at all: lemons, green apples, sour salads – in other words, purely things with little nutritional value and few calories. In addition, such patients generally use aperients or laxatives in order to get rid of what little they eat just as surely and quickly as they can. They also have a strong need for physical exercise. They go for long walks to work off the fat that they never put on in the first place – an activity which in the light of their often weakened condition is little short of astonishing. At the same time such patients are remarkable for their exaggerated altruism: this quite often culminates in their actually being willing to cook for others, which they will do with great conscientiousness. The fact of cooking for others, acting as their hosts and looking after them while they eat worries them not a jot, as long as they do not have to join in themselves. And yet despite all this they have a real yen for solitude, and tend to be reclusive. Frequently the menstrual periods of female anorexics stop altogether, or at least they have problems and disturbances in this area.

Summing up the symptomatology, then, what we have here is an exaggeration of the ascetic ideal. Underlying it all is the old conflict between spirit and matter, above and below, purity and animal instinct. The job of food is to build up the body and so nourish the world of forms. When anorexics say 'no' to food, what they are really saying 'no' to is physicality and all the demands of the body. The real ideal of anorexics goes far beyond the sphere of mere food: their aim is purity and spiritualisation. Their desire is to free themselves from the weight of the body entirely. They are concerned to escape all sexuality and instinct. Their goal is chastity and sexlessness. This necessarily involves staying as slim as possible, for otherwise bulges are liable to appear on the body which will reveal that the anorexic in question is a woman – which is precisely what she has no wish to be.

The rounded female form is not the only thing that such patients are afraid of: a fat belly also reminds them of the possibility of getting pregnant. Their resistance to their own femininity and sexuality therefore also manifests itself in a failure of their monthly periods. The highest ideal of anorexics is dematerialisation – to stay clear of everything that has anything to do with base physicality.

In the light of this ascetic ideal, anorexics do not classify themselves as ill at all, and fail totally to understand all the various therapeutic treatments which only go to serve the body from which they are so anxious to distance themselves. And so they cleverly get around every attempt to force-feed them in hospital by using more and more sophisticated tricks to dispose of all the food on the sly. They reject all help, and determinedly pursue their ideal of leaving all corporeal considerations behind them by spiritualising everything. Death is not seen as a threat at all – for it is precisely the world of the living that produces so much fear in them. They are afraid of everything that is rounded, amorphous, feminine, fertile, instinctive and sexual – and so they are afraid of intimacy and warmth, too. It is for this reason that anorexics will not join in communal meals. Sitting around a table breaking bread together is in all cultures a time-honoured ritual that gives rise to human intimacy and warmth. Yet it is precisely this intimacy that fills anorexics with such fear.

This fear draws its nourishment from their shadow-world, in which all the themes that have been so carefully avoided on the conscious level are lurking, eagerly awaiting their chance to make their presence felt. Anorexics have an enormous craving for life – a craving which they then use their symptomatic behaviour to try and eradicate, out of fear of being totally overwhelmed by it all. Yet from time to time they find themselves overtaken by the very craving and greed that they are so anxious to resist and repress. And so the secret bingeing starts. Out of feelings of guilt this 'slip' is then made good again by vomiting. Thus, anorexics never succeed in finding a happy medium in the conflict between greed and asceticism, between hunger and renunciation, between self-centredness and self-sacrifice. Behind altruistic behaviour there is always to be found a thickly-veiled egocentricity, which soon becomes only too apparent when dealing with such patients. They have a secret longing for attention, and exact it by being ill. Those who refuse to eat have at their immediate disposal undreamt-of power over other people, who in their anxiety and despair assume that it is somehow their job to make them eat again and so survive. Even small children use this trick to rule their families with a rod of iron.

There is no way in which anorexics can be helped by force-feeding them: the most one can do is to help them to be honest with themselves. Patients have to discover and accept their own greed, their craving for love and sex, their egocentricity and their femininity, with all the instinctiveness and corporeality that this entails. They have to grasp the fact that the earthly realm is not to be outgrown either by resistance or by repression, but only by integrating it, living it out for real and thereby transmuting it. In the light of this fact there are a good many of us who could well learn a lesson from the symptomatology of anorexia. Anorexics are not the only ones who tend to use sophisticated-sounding philosophical arguments in order to repress the disturbing claims of their own physicality and live 'clean', 'spiritual' lives. It is all too easy to overlook the fact that ascetism generally throws a shadow – and that the name of that shadow is . . . greed.

Five

The Sense Organs

The sense organs are the portals of our awareness. It is through the sense organs that we are connected with the outside world. They are the windows of our soul through which we eventually perceive ... ourselves. For in fact the outer world that we perceive with our senses, and in whose incontestable reality we believe so firmly, does not really exist at all.

Let us endeavour to explain this sweeping assertion step by step. How does our process of perception work? Every act of sensual perception can be reduced to a piece of information that comes into being as a result of changes in vibration at the particle-level. Looking at an iron rod, for example, we can see its black colour, detect the coldness of the metal, smell its characteristic smell and feel how hard it is. If we now heat up the iron rod with a Bunsen burner, we notice how the colour alters as it starts to glow red, we can feel the heat that it is emitting, we can test out and see for ourselves its new plasticity. What has happened? We have merely applied energy to the iron rod, as a result of which the velocity of its particles has increased. This increased particle-velocity has in turn led to changes in perception which we then describe in terms of the words 'red', 'hot', 'flexible' and so on.

We can see clearly from this example how our entire perceptual process rests upon particle-vibrations and upon changes in their frequency. The particles impinge on specific receptors in our sense organs, triggering reactions in them which in turn are transmitted in the form of electrochemical impulses via the nervous system to the brain, where a complex image is produced which we then go on to call 'red', 'smelly' and so on. What goes in, then, is particles: what comes out is complex perceptual patterns – and in between the two lies only our own processing. And yet we still imagine that the complex images that our consciousness puts together on the basis of the original particle-data really exist independently of ourselves! This is where our error lies. 'Out there', in fact, there is nothing but particles – yet it is precisely these that we have never succeeded in actually perceiving at all. Granted that our entire perception rests on particles, we still cannot perceive those particles. In reality, then, we are surrounded only by our own subjective images. True, we assume that other people (do they really exist?) perceive the same things as we do, in view of the fact that they use the same words for what they perceive – and yet no two people can ever establish whether they are actually seeing the same thing when they use the word 'green'. We are for ever totally alone, surrounded by our own images – and yet we make the most strenuous efforts to avoid facing up to this truth.

All these images have just the same validity – exactly the same validity, in fact – as dream images have, at least so long as we are still dreaming them. One day, though, we shall awake out of our persistent daydream to discover that the world which we imagine to be so real has dissolved into nothingness – into *maya*, illusion, a mere veil that hangs between us and reality. Anyone who has followed our argument thus far may of course object that, even though the outer world may admittedly not exist as we perceive it, *some* kind of 'outer world' must exist, even if it only consists of particles. Yet even this notion is deceptive. For on the particle-level there is no longer any detectable distinction between 'I' and 'not-I', between 'inner' and 'outer'. There is no way of telling from a particle whether it is part of myself or of the world around me. At this level there are no frontiers. Here all is One.

That, indeed, is precisely what is meant by the ancient esoteric teaching: 'Microcosm = macrocosm'. The equals-sign applies here with all its mathematical exactness. The 'I', or ego, is an illusion, an artificial boundary that exists only in the mind – at least, that is, until we have learnt to give up the 'I', only to discover to our astonishment that the *aloneness* which we fear so much is really an *all-one-ness*. Yet the route to this oneness – the path of *at-one-ment* – is long and wearisome. All that binds us to the perceived world of matter is our five senses – just as Jesus himself was nailed by his five wounds to the cross of the material world. But this cross can be overcome only by taking it upon ourselves and turning it into a vehicle of the 'rebirth in the spirit'.

We said at the beginning of this chapter that the sense organs are the windows of our soul through which we perceive ourselves. That which we call the environment or outer world is in fact a series of reflections of our soul. A mirror enables us to observe and recognise ourselves better, because it also shows us those areas of ourselves which we are unable to see at all other than via their reflections. Thus the apparent world around us is the most marvellous of aids on our route to self-knowledge. Since what we see in this mirror is not always very pleasing – for our shadow, too, is to be seen in it – we are very much concerned to distinguish between ourselves and what is 'out there', so that we can insist that whatever it is 'has nothing to do with me'. But therein lies our danger. We project our essence 'out there' and then believe in the independence of that projection. Then we neglect to take the projection back again – and so the time for 'social work' begins, with all of us helping everybody else but none of us bothering to help ourselves. True, to help us on our way towards self-knowledge we need to see our reflection in the 'outer world'. Yet we should not neglect to reabsorb our projections into ourselves if we ever want to become whole again. Jewish mythology puts this point across via the imagery of the creation of woman. From the complete, androgynous man who is Adam, one side (the old translations use the word 'rib') is removed and fashioned into something that is formally independent. From this point onwards, then, Adam lacks one half of himself, which he then proceeds to encounter as his 'opposite half'. He has become *un-whole*, and can only become whole again by uniting himself with that which he is now lacking. Yet this can only happen by way of the outer world. If during the course of our lives we neglect gradually to reintegrate the perceived 'outer world' – thanks to having given in to the enticing illusion that what is happening 'out there' has 'nothing to do with us' – then our consequent destiny will gradually start to get in the way of any growth in our awareness.

'Awareness' consists in taking full account of the truth. This can only happen to the extent that we recognise ourselves in everything that we perceive. If we forget this, the windows of our soul that are our sense organs gradually grow dim and opaque and so force us finally to direct our perception inwards. The measure in which the sense organs cease to work properly is thus the same measure in which we ourselves are taught to look within, to listen within, to hear what is going on inside us. We are forced to 'reflect upon ourselves', and so to 'come to our senses' once more.

Indeed, there are specific meditation techniques which enable us spontaneously to 'come to our senses'. Using the fingers of both hands to close the gates of awareness – the ears, the eyes and the mouth – subjects meditate on the corresponding inner sense-impressions, which after a certain amount of practice manifest themselves as ... sound, colour and taste.

The Eyes

The eyes do not merely let sense-impressions in – they also let something out; for in them we can see a person's moods and feelings. That is why we search the eyes of others, trying to look into them and read what they have to say. The eyes are the mirrors of the soul. It is the eyes, similarly, that break out in tears and so reveal outwardly what is happening to the psyche inwardly. True, iridology has so far used the eyes purely as a mirror of the body, yet it is just as possible to read a person's character and personality make-up from their eyes. A 'dirty look' or the 'evil eye' likewise show that the eye is not just an organ for letting things in, but can also let out what is inside us. Again, the eyes are used in an active way when we 'throw a glance' at somebody. Self-love is also often referred to as 'self-regard' – an expression which immediately reveals that those concerned can no longer see reality clearly: in such circumstances, after all, it is all too easy for them to get the wrong impression of themselves, for 'love is blind' – even if the fact doesn't immediately 'strike the eye'!

The most common conditions that affect the eye are short-sightedness and long-sightedness – of which short-sightedness mainly affects young people and long-sightedness is an affliction of old age. This division is of obvious relevance, since young people tend for the most part to be aware only of their own immediate environment, and therefore to be lacking in perspective and depth of vision. Old people, by contrast, are better able to stand back and take the longer view. In the same way old people's memories show not just a tendency to forget quite recent events, but an outstanding ability to recall long-past events in astonishing detail.

Short-sightedness is a sign of too much subjectivity. People who are short-sighted see everything exclusively 'through their own eyes' – or, as the Germans put it, 'through their own glasses' (*durch eigene Brille*) – and thus take everything personally. They 'can see no further than the end of their noses' – yet even so this restricted range of vision still fails to lead them to self-knowledge. This is where the real problem lies – for we certainly need to relate everything we see to ourselves if ever we are to get to know ourselves. Yet this process degenerates into its opposite the moment it gets bogged down in subjectivity. What this amounts to in practice is that those involved do indeed relate everything to themselves, but then refuse to see or to recognise themselves in it. Their subjective approach merely leads to an attitude of injured innocence or to some other defensive reaction, with the projection never actually being unmasked for what it is at all.

Short-sightedness exposes this misunderstanding. It forces us to look more closely at what intimately concerns us. It brings our point of sharpest vision closer to our own eyes, nearer to the tip of our own noses. In the process, short-sightedness shows in bodily form our high degree of subjectivity, and by the same token promotes self-knowledge. For true self-knowledge necessarily leads us out of our subjectivity. If we cannot see (or, at best, see poorly) then the operative question is: 'What is it that I don't *want* to see?' The answer is always: 'Myself.'

The extent of our refusal to look at ourselves in this way can easily be gauged merely from the refractive index of whatever glasses we are prescribed. Spectacles are a prosthesis and by the same token a deception. We use them artifically to offset an entirely reasonable adjustment to our circumstances, and then act as though everything were still perfectly in order. This deception is increased considerably by the wearing of contact-lenses, in that they enable us to hush up even the fact that we 'cannot see very well'. Imagine, then, what would happen if we were to take away everybody's glasses and contact-lenses overnight. Suddenly we would all realise just how people actually view the world and – more to the point – would be able to experience the extent of our own inability to see things as they are. (To be of any use to us, after all, a handicap needs to be experienced *personally*.) All of a sudden we should all have a chance to *real-ise* just how 'unclear' our view of the world is, how 'blurred' our sight and how restricted our vision. Perhaps 'the scales would fall from our eyes' – for some of us, at least – and we should start to see things in a clearer light, for how can we hope to attain true *in-sight* if we cannot even see properly in the first place?

On the basis of their experience of life, meanwhile, old people should have developed wisdom and far-sightedness. Unfortunately, however, many of them manifest this far-sightedness only on the physical level, in the form of *long*-sightedness. By contrast, *colour-blindness* reveals to us our blindness to all life's colour and variety. People who suffer from it see everything in shades of grey and are anxious to iron out all distinctions – in a word, they tend to be colourless people.

Like all inflammatory conditions, *conjunctivitis* speaks to us of conflict. It leads to pain in the eyes which can be eased only by shutting them. Sufferers are thus closing their eyes to some conflict so as not to look it in the face.

Squinting: When viewing things we need two images in order to be able to see them in their full dimensionality. Who can fail to recognise in this statement the whole law of polarity all over again? We always need two ways of seeing to appreciate any entity in its entirety. If, however, the axes of our vision are not co-ordinated with each other, the result is a squint – the retinas of our two eyes receive two incongruent images (double vision). Lest we should actually *see* two divergent images, though, the brain 'makes up its mind' to filter out one of the two images entirely (namely the image formed in the squinting eye). As a result we virtually become one-eyed, since the image formed in the second eye is not transmitted any further. We see everything as flat, and so lose all sense of dimensionality.

It is just the same with polarity itself. Here, too, we have to be able to see both poles as a single image (for example, waves *and* particles, free will *and* predestination, good *and* evil). If we cannot manage this and the two images consequently appear to clash with one another, we switch off one of the two ways of seeing (by repressing it) and so become one-eyed rather than single-sighted. Those of us who squint are truly one-eyed, in that the image of the second eye is suppressed by the brain, so leading to a loss of dimensionality and a consequently 'one-sided' outlook.

Cataract: In the case of a cataract the lens becomes cloudy – and consequently our vision becomes cloudy too. We can no longer see things sharply. For all our failure to 'see things sharply', however, they still have 'sharp edges' – they can injure us for all that. Yet to the extent that we blunt this dangerous sharpness by blurring its image, our world, too, seems to lose all danger of injury. Fuzzy vision corresponds to a reassuring distancing of ourselves from the world around us – and therefore also from our real selves. A cataract is rather like a 'blind' that we pull down in order not to have to see what we would rather not see. It covers our eyes like scales – and indeed can lead to blindness.

Glaucoma: With glaucoma, raised pressure within the eye leads to an increasing restriction of the field of vision until actual tunnel vision results. Patients see the world as though through blinkers. The wider view is lost to sight – in effect, they are blind to all except that one aspect of reality that they *want* to see. And behind it all lies the psychological stress of unwept tears (as expressed by the raised pressure within the eye).

Blindness: This is the most extreme form of not wanting to see. To most people, losing one's sight is perhaps the most grievous of all losses that can befall the body. Metaphorically, too, we use the expression 'He was struck blind' in a similarly catastrophic sense. For blind people the external projection-screen is finally taken away and so they are forced to look inwards. Physical blindness is merely the ultimate manifestation of the blindness that is really at issue – namely, blindness of consciousness.

A few years back a number of young blind people in the USA were given back their sight thanks to a new surgical technique. The outcome was by no means all joy and gladness, however. Indeed, most of those operated on found themselves unable to adjust to the change or come to grips with the normal world again. Naturally we can try to analyse and explain this phenomenon from a number of angles. From our own point of view, however, the sole point of any importance is that mechanical measures, while admittedly capable of changing physical functions themselves, cannot remove the basic problems of which the symptoms are merely manifestations. Only when we finally stop looking at every handicap as an unwelcome disturbance to be removed or compensated for as quickly and as unobtrusively as possible are we likely to gain anything from the disturbance. It is actually important for us to let the disturbance disturb our normal way of life: our job is to *let* it stop us carrying on living as we have been hitherto. In this way illness can turn into a path that leads us to healing. In this way, too, even blindness can teach us true vision and lead us on to deeper insight.

EYE PROBLEMS

Should you have problems with your eyes or your vision, the first step is to put aside your glasses (or contact-lenses) for a whole day so as consciously to experience the totally unvarnished life-situation that results. At the end of the day, make a written account of just how you saw and experienced things, what you could and could not do, what you found difficult, how you coped with those around you and so on. Such an account should provide you with plenty of material for getting to know yourself and those around you a good deal better. Basically you should also look into the following questions:

1. What is it that I do not *want* to see?
2. Is my subjectivity getting in the way of my self-awareness?
3. Am I neglecting to recognise myself in everything that happens?
4. Am I really using my vision to further my insight?
5. Am I afraid to see things in their full clarity?
6. Can I really bear to see things as they are at all?
7. Which aspect of my nature is it that I am so keen to look away from?

The Ears

Let us first of all listen in once again to a few common idioms and turns of speech in which we refer to the ears or hearing. To 'keep our ears open' – to 'lend someone an ear' – to 'give somebody a hearing' – to 'harken to someone' – 'Do you hear?' – 'Hear us, O Lord!' – 'Now hear this!' All these expressions reveal a clear link between the ears and the idea of letting in, of 'being passive' (harkening) and thus eventually of obedience. Compared with our hearing, sight is a much more active form of perception. For this reason it is also much easier actively to look away or to shut our eyes to things than it is to close our ears. Our capacity for hearing is a bodily expression of how obedient and submissive we are. Thus it is that we sometimes ask a disobedient child, 'Are you deaf?' Those who are hard of hearing are people who will not listen. They simply fail to hear what they do not want to hear. It shows a certain egocentricity to refuse to lend an ear to others or take anything on board any more. It shows a lack of submissiveness, of willingness to 'harken' or obey. This is precisely what happens in the case of noise-induced deafness. It is not the sheer volume of noise that does the damage, but the psychological resistance to the noise: *not wanting* to let it in leads to *not being able* to let it in. The frequent ear-inflammations and earaches suffered by children occur predominantly at an age when they are having to learn obedience. Most old people, for their part, are smitten by hardness of hearing to a certain degree. Such hardness of hearing belongs, like poor sight, stiffness and immobility, to the physical symptoms of old age, which are all expressions of our tendency to become more and more rigid and inflexible with age. Most old people lose their adaptability and flexibility and become ever more *unwilling to listen*. Although the picture just outlined is typical of the development of old people, it is of course in no way *de rigueur*. Age merely exaggerates those problems that have not yet been resolved, and makes us just as honest as does illness itself.

As for 'auditory collapse', this is a sudden, mainly unilateral, severe impairment of hearing or even deafness originating in the inner ear, which may later spread to the other ear as well. In order to interpret it, it is important to look closely at the actual life-situation in which it arises. Auditory collapse is a summons to listen to what is going on inside us and harken to our own inner voice. If we go deaf, it is only because we have long since 'turned a deaf ear' to the voice within.

EAR PROBLEMS

In the event of problems with your ears or hearing, you would do well to ask yourself:

1. Why am I not prepared to lend other people an ear?
2. Who or what am I refusing to listen to?
3. Are the two poles of self-centredness and submissiveness in a good state of balance within me?

Headaches

Headaches were unknown until only a few centuries ago: in earlier cultural epochs they were unheard of. It is particularly in civilised countries that headaches have been on the rise in recent years, with 20 per cent of 'healthy people' claiming to suffer from them. Statistics show that women are afflicted somewhat more frequently, and that the 'upper classes', too, are 'over-represented' as far as this symptom is concerned. Once we get around to 'cudgelling our brains' about the symbolism of the head, though, we discover that there is little to surprise us in all this. The head stands in a clear polar relationship to the body. It 'heads' our whole bodily 'organisation'. It is what maintains our head-ing for us. The head represents the Above, just as the body expresses the Below.

We normally regard the head as the place where understanding, reason and thought have their abode. People who are 'off their heads' are not reasonable people. We can 'turn a person's head' but we should not then expect them to 'keep a cool head' in the process. Feelings as irrational as love naturally 'go to our heads' – indeed most people 'lose their heads' completely over it (and if not, they finish up with a 'sore head'!). But then we also have a few 'headstrong' contemporaries who somehow manage to 'keep their heads on their shoulders' even when 'running their heads against a brick wall'. Some observers venture to explain this by describing them as 'blockheads' – but unfortunately this cannot be scientifically confirmed one way or the other.

Tension headache starts out as a semi-acute, diffuse pain in the head, generally of an oppressive kind, which can drag on for hours, days or even weeks. The pain involved seems to be the result of too high a pressure in the blood-vessels. Generally speaking, tension-headache is simultaneously accompanied by a powerful tensing of the musculature of the head, as well as of the muscles in the area of the shoulders, the neck and the cervical vertebrae. Quite frequently tension-headaches arise when people are subjected to over-heavy work pressures, or in critical situations involving promotion that threaten to over-extend them.

It is the 'way upwards' that can so easily lead to an over emphasis of the upper pole – and thus of the head. Behind the symptomatology of headaches we often find proud perfectionists who are attempting to enforce their own will (and 'running their heads against a brick wall' in the process). In such cases it is all too easy for pride and power-mania to 'go to their heads', for if we pay attention only to the world of the head, and are prepared to accept and live out only what is rational, reasonable and understandable, we soon lose our connection with the 'lower pole' and thus with our roots, which alone are capable of giving us a real footing in life. We become 'top-heavy'. Yet the claims of the body and its mostly unconscious functions have a much longer evolutionary pedigree than our capacity for rational thought, which – along with the development of the cerebral cortex – represents a later human achievement altogether.

As human beings we have two main centres: the heart and the brain – feeling and thinking. Modern human culture has developed the brain's powers to a considerable degree and is therefore in constant danger of neglecting the other centre that is the heart. But equally it is no solution immediately to denigrate thought, reason and the head generally. Neither aspect is any better or worse than the other. It is not for us to decide in favour of the one or against the other. Our job is to strive for balance.

Thus, those who are 'bottom-heavy' are just as *un-whole* as those who are 'top-heavy'. And yet our culture has promoted the development of the head-pole so strongly that most of us are deficient where the lower pole is concerned.

The further problem then arises as to what we use our intellectual activity *for*. By and large we apply our capacity for rational thought to assuring and guaranteeing our 'I'. With the aid of causal thinking we do our best to insure ourselves increasingly against what fate has in store for us, with the aim of extending our ego-dominance even further. Yet any such undertaking is in the last resort bound to end in failure. As in the case of the Tower of Babel, it can lead only to confusion. It is simply not 'on' for the head to declare its independence and pursue a path of its own without the body or the heart. The moment thinking cuts itself off from below it lets go of its roots. Science's purely rationalist way of thinking is an example of this rootlessness, for it lacks all connection with the original source – with all *religio*. Those of us who only follow our heads rise to ever dizzier heights without ever being anchored to what lies below – in which case it is little wonder if we find 'our heads in a swim'. For it is our heads, in the event, that actually sound the alarm.

Of all parts of our bodies, it is our heads that are quickest to react with pain. In all our internal organs much more thorough-going changes have to occur before pain arises. The head is our most sensitive alarm-system. When it aches, it is a sure sign that our thinking has gone off the rails, that we are applying our thought wrongly, that we are pursuing dubious ends. It sounds the alarm as soon as we start 'worrying our heads' with pointless broodings over all kinds of non-existent certainties. Within the context of our material existence there is absolutely nothing that we can ever guarantee – indeed, every attempt to do so merely turns us into a laughing-stock.

We are always cudgelling our brains about total non-essentials – to the point where 'our heads start buzzing'. Releasing that tension is a matter of relaxing – but then this is merely another word for letting go. As soon as a headache sounds the alarm, it is high time that we let go of our narrow-minded self-interest, of all the pride that is driving us ever on-ward and upward, of all our stubbornness and 'pig-headedness'. It is high time, too, that we directed our gaze downwards and started to contemplate our roots. There is no help for those who smother all such warning notes for years on end with pain-killers: they are merely 'risking their necks' and 'laying their heads on the block'.

Migraine

According to Braütigam,

> Migraine (hemicrania) consists of a sudden and for the most part lateralised headache which may be accompanied by visual disturbances (such as sensitivity to light or flickering) along with added stomach or digestive components such as vomiting or diarrhoea. Generally lasting several hours, the attack has its roots in a depressive and sensitive disposition. The climax of a migraine attack produces an urgent wish to be alone and to withdraw to some dark room or to bed.

In contrast to tension-headaches, migraines produce initial spasms followed by considerable dilatation of the blood-vessels in the brain. The Greek for migraine, *hemikrania (kranion =*

'cranium'), literally means 'half-headedness' and points directly towards the one-sided thinking that is to be found in just the same form in migraine patients as in tension-headache cases.

Everything that we have said in this latter connection applies equally to migraine, but it needs to be modified in one basic respect. Whereas sufferers from tension-headaches are trying to separate their heads from their bodies, migraine-patients are transferring one particular bodily theme into their heads and trying to live it out at this level instead. That theme is sexuality. Migraine is always a displacement of sexuality into the head. The head is reassigned what is really the body's job. In fact this particular displacement is not as irrelevant as all that, for the genital area and head stand in an analogical relationship to each other. They are, after all, the two parts of the body that contain all the bodily orifices.

The part played by the bodily orifices in sexuality is of course an absolutely vital one (love, in the sense of 'letting in', can after all only be realised at the physical level at those points where the body is capable of opening itself up). Common parlance has long associated a woman's mouth with her vagina (take the case of 'dry lips', for example) and a man's nose with his penis, and has sought to draw inferences from the one to the other. In the case of oral intercourse, too, this relationship – this 'interchangeability' – between head and body is patently obvious. Head and body are polarities, and behind their opposition stands their common identity: as Above, so Below. Just how frequently the head is used to stand in for the body is something that can readily be seen from the phenomenon of blushing. In embarrassing situations, which nearly always have a background connotation that is more or less sexual in charac-ter, the blood goes to our head and makes it go red. In the process, what should really be happening 'down below' is manifested at the higher level – for normally sexual excitement causes the blood to flow to the genital area, making the sexual organs swell up and go red. We find the same transference from the genital area to the head in cases of impotence. The more a man's thoughts are in his head during sexual intercourse, the more likely he is to lose potency at the bodily level – with embarrassing consequences. A similar transference is applied by sexually frustrated people who eat more and more by way of compensation. A good many of us try to satisfy our hunger for love by way of our mouths – and naturally never feel full up. All these indications should suffice to draw our attention to the analogy that exists between lower body and head. Migraine patients (more often women than men) always have problems with their sexuality.

As we have already emphasised several times in other connections, there are basically two ways of coping with any given problem area. Either we can push it away from us and repress it ('nip it in the bud') or we can dramatically over-compensate for it. The two approaches may seem to be very different, yet they are no more than polar expressions of a single difficulty. When we are afraid, we may either quake in our boots or flay about us wildly – yet both reactions are expressions of weakness. In just the same way we find among migraine patients both people who have banished their sexuality totally from their lives ('I don't have anything to do with such things') and people who are anxious to impress on everybody what a marvellous sex-life they have. It is all one: both kinds have problems with their sexuality. Refusing to admit to this problem, either because we insist that sex has 'nothing to do with us' or because 'anybody can see for themselves that we just don't *have* any sex-problems', merely forces the problem into our heads, where it reappears as migraine. At which point we can set about working on the problem at a higher level.

A migraine attack is in some ways like an orgasm in the head. What happens is similar in both cases: it is just that its site lies higher up. Just as sexual excitement causes the blood to flow to the genital region and the tension reverts to relaxation at the climax, so it is with migraine: blood flows to the head, there is a feeling of pressure, the tension increases and then changes back suddenly to relaxation (dilatation of the blood-vessels). Any stimulus, anything that arouses us, can produce a migraine attack – light, noise, stress, weather, excitement and so on. And it is indeed one of migraine's characteristic traits that for some time after the attack patients enjoy a distinct feeling of well-being. Moreover, at the climax of the attack they would much prefer to be in bed in a dark room – though in this case alone.

All this shows the essentially sexual nature of what is involved, as well as the fear of working out the relevant problem with somebody else on the appropriate level. As early as 1934, E. Gutheil described in a psychoanalytical periodical a patient whose migraine attacks ceased after sexual orgasm. Sometimes several orgasms were necessary before relaxation set in and the attack came to an end. It is also relevant to our enquiry that digestive disturbances and constipation are high on the list of migraine patients' side-symptoms: in other words such people are 'closed up' at the lower level. They do not want to catch sight of their own unconscious contents (their excrement) and therefore retreat upwards into conscious thought – until 'their heads are buzzing'. Married couples also tend to use their migraines (quite often the word merely refers to a common-or-garden headache) as an excuse for not having sex.

To sum up, then, we find in migraine patients a conflict between instinct and thought, between Below and Above, which leads to an attempt to use the head as a bolt-hole, and as a workout-area for trying to solve problems which can in fact only be expressed and resolved on other levels entirely (body, sex, aggression). Even Freud described thinking as an experimental activity. We tend to regard thought as less dangerous and less committed than action itself. Yet the function of thought is not to replace action: instead, the one has to support the other. We have been given a body as a tool for *real-ising* ourselves. Only through this realisation can our various energies continue to flow. It is thus no accident that terms such as 'understanding' and 'grasping' evoke highly physical images. Our understanding and our ability to grasp things are rooted in our use of our feet and hands – of our body. Any breaking-up of this team-activity leads to increasingly solid blockages of energy which go on to manifest themselves as illness, in the form of a variety of groups of symptoms. The following review may help to illustrate this point:

Degrees of Escalation of Blocked Energy

1. If activity such as sex or aggression is blocked at the *mental* level, the result is headaches.
2. If the activity is blocked at the *vegetative* level (at the level of the autonomous body-functions) this leads to high blood-pressure and the symptomatology of vegetative dystonia.
3. If the activity is blocked at the *neurological* level, this leads to a symptomatology such as that of multiple sclerosis.
4. If the activity is restricted at the *muscular* level, we encounter problems of the motor system, such as rheumatism or arthritis.

This phase-division corresponds closely to the various phases of what would actually have happened in practice. Every activity – be it a mere punch or actual sexual intercourse – begins (1) with a conceptual phase, in which the activity is anticipated mentally. This leads (2) to the vegetative preparation of the body, in the form of increased blood-supply to the particular organs involved, raised pulse-rate and so on. Finally the thought is transmitted (3) via the nerves (4) to the muscles, which translate it into action. Whenever a thought is not translated into action, the associated energy is inevitably blocked in one of the four areas involved (thought, vegetative system, nerves or muscles) and in time produces corresponding symptoms in that area.

Migraine patients are on the first rung of this ladder: they are blocking their sexuality at the conceptual phase. They need to learn to see their problem for what it is, so as to restore what has 'gone to their heads' to where it belongs – down below. Development always starts at the bottom, and the way up is long and demanding – always assuming that we pursue it honestly.

HEADACHES

In the event of headache or migraine, ask yourself the following questions:

1. What am I 'worrying my head about'?
2. Are 'above' and 'below' still actively working together within me?
3. Am I trying too hard to work my way up? Am I suffering from an excess of pride?
4. Am I pig-headed, and trying to 'run my head against a brick wall'?
5. Am I trying to replace doing with thinking?
6. Am I facing my sexual problems honestly?
7. Why am I pushing my orgasm into my head?

Seven

The Skin

The skin is the largest human organ. It fulfils a variety of functions, of which the most important are as follows:

1. Separation and protection
2. Touch and contact
3. Expression and representation
4. Sexuality
5. Respiration
6. Excretion (sweat)
7. Temperature-regulation.

All these diverse skin-functions nevertheless have a common theme that hovers between the two poles of separation and contact. For us, the skin is our outermost physical boundary, and yet at the same time it connects us to the outside world and brings us into contact with our environment. It is via our skin that we present ourselves to the world . . . and we *cannot change our skins*. The skin reflects our nature externally – and in a very simple way, at that. For a start, it serves as a reflective surface for all our internal organs. Every disturbance of those organs is projected onto the skin, and every stimulation of the corresponding skin-area is transmitted back inwards to the organ in question. This link is the basis of all the various 'reflex-zone therapies' that have long been used in natural healing, even though only a very few of them are currently applied in academic medicine (as in the case of the so-called 'Head' zones). Of particular note here are reflexology's foot-zone massage, the use of 'cupping' in connection with the dorsal zones, nasal reflexology and aural acupuncture (to name but a few).

The experienced practitioner is capable of seeing and feeling from the skin the condition of the various organs, and equally of treating these organs via their particular projection-sites on the skin.

Whatever happens to the skin – a reddening, a swelling, an inflammation, a spot, an abscess – the site of this occurrence is no accident, but refers to a corresponding inner process. Time was when there were sophisticated systems for telling the character of a person from the positions of their moles, for example. The Age of Enlightenment duly threw such 'patent nonsense' overboard as sheer superstition – yet we are gradually working our way back towards an understanding of these things. Is it really so very hard to grasp, after all, that behind the whole of creation there stands an invisible pattern which merely *expresses* itself via the physical realm? Everything visible is merely a likeness of the invisible, just as a work of art is the visible expression of the invisible idea in the mind of the artist. From the visible we make inferences about the invisible. This is something that we all do the whole time, even in our everyday life. We go into somebody's living-room and on the basis of what we see there draw conclusions about the taste of the person who lives there. But we could have diagnosed the self-same taste by looking into that person's wardrobe. *Where* we look is a matter of total indifference – if a person has bad taste (or whatever) this will show in everything that he or she touches.

And so the entire information pattern constantly manifests itself everywhere at once. In every part we find the whole (the Romans referred to this relationship in the words *pars pro toto*). That is why it is of no importance which part of a person's body we look at. The same pattern is to be seen everywhere – the particular pattern, that is to say, which the person in question represents. We can find this pattern in the eye (iridology), in the ear (French aural acupuncture), in the back, in the feet, in the meridian-points (terminal-point diagnosis), in every drop of blood (crystallisation-testing, capillardynamolysis, holistic blood-diagnosis), in every body-cell (human genetics), in the hand (chirology), in the face and physical build (physiognomy), and of course in the skin (the subject currently under consideration).

The aim of this book is to help us get to know ourselves as human beings through our symptoms. It makes not a jot of difference where we look – always provided that we know *how* to look. The truth is omnipresent. If only the specialists were to let go of their obsession with trying to demonstrate the causality underlying all the various connections that they have discovered, they would suddenly see that everything stands in an analogical relationship to everything else. As Above, so Below; as within, so without.

Yet the skin does not merely reveal our internal organic state: on and within it are also to be seen all our psychological processes and reactions. In some respects this is so apparent that we can all see it for ourselves: we go red with embarrassment and pale with shock, we sweat with fear or excitement, our hair bristles with horror or we get gooseflesh. Outwardly invisible, meanwhile, yet still measurable with the aid of suitable electronic equipment, is the skin's electrical conductivity. The original experiments and measurements in this area go right back to C. G. Jung, who explored this area in connection with his experiments into psychological association techniques. Thanks to modern electronics, it is possible today to display the continual fine alterations in skin-conductivity and to enhance them to such an extent that it is possible to 'interrogate' a person purely via their skin, for every word, every subject, every question draws forth a response from the skin in the form of an immediate fine adjustment in its electrical activity (the so-called electro-galvanic skin response).

All of which goes to confirm that the skin is nothing so much as a great projection screen on which not only physical, but psychological processes and happenings are constantly made visible. But then, if the skin reveals so much of what is going on inside us, it is but a short step to start thinking in terms not only of looking after it, but actually of manipulating what it looks like. This fraudulent undertaking is what we refer to as 'cosmetics', and we are quite willing to invest princely sums in this deceptive art. It is not our intention here to create a song and dance about the cosmetic arts or about self-beautification generally, but we do propose to take a look at just what kind of human endeavour it is that underlies the age-old tradition of body-painting. If the skin is the outward expression of what is going on inside us, then every attempt artificially to alter that expression is necessarily an act of dishonesty. We are either trying to hush something up, or else making a pretence at something. If we are making a pretence at something, then it is because that 'something' isn't really there inside us at all. We build up a false façade, and so the correspondence between form and content goes by the board. What we run up against here, in short, is the difference between 'being beautiful' and 'looking beautiful', between reality and appearance. This effort to show a false face to the world starts with simple make-up and finishes in such grotesque guises as cosmetic surgery. Those concerned actually have their faces 'lifted'. How strange it is that people are so unafraid to 'lose face' in this way!

Behind all these attempts to become other than we are lies the basic problem that we like nobody less than ourselves. To love ourselves is one of the sternest challenges facing us. Those of us who imagine that they do love themselves are assuredly mixing up the idea of 'self' with their own tiny egos. The only people who think that they like themselves are people who do not yet know who they are. It is precisely because we do *not* like ourselves (inclusive of our shadow) that we are constantly trying to alter and mould our external image. Yet this remains purely cosmetic all the while the inner person – or rather that person's consciousness – does not change. (At the same time, though, we would not dream of questioning the possibility that changes of form can help initiate an inwardly orientated process, much as happens in hatha yoga, bionergetics and similar approaches. What differentiates such methods from cosmetics is the subject's consciousness of the goal to be attained!) Even on mere passing acquaintance, people's skin tells us a good deal about their psyche. Beneath a highly sensitive skin there lies a highly sensitive soul (in other words they are people with 'thin skins'), while a tough, resistant skin tends rather to suggest someone who is 'thick-skinned'. A sweaty skin reveals insecurity and fear vis-à-vis those around us, a reddening of the skin excitement. It is with the skin that we touch and come into contact with others. Whether in the case of a punch or of gentle stroking, it is always the skin that establishes direct contact between us. When we are ill, the skin can be broken through either from inside (inflammation, rash, abscess) or from outside (injury, operation). In both cases our limits are compromised, and we may not even succeed in 'saving our skins'.

Skin Rashes

In the case of a skin rash, something is bursting through our limits – something that needs to get out. It is easiest to see this point in connection with the typical acne of puberty. At puberty it is human sexuality that is trying to break out, but at the same time it is for the most part anxiously repressed in the very attempt to do so. Puberty is an excellent example of a conflict-situation. In the midst of a phase of apparent calm a totally new impulse suddenly breaks forth out of the depths of the unconscious, and strives with all its strength to make space for itself in the young person's life and consciousness. But this new thing that is making its presence felt is unknown and unfamiliar, and induces great fear. There is a strong urge to expunge it again and return once more to the old, familiar state of affairs. Yet this is just not 'on' anymore. You cannot make a trend *un*-happen.

And so the young people concerned are up to their ears in conflict. The thrill of the new and the fear of the new tug at them with almost equal force. Every conflict follows the same pattern. It is merely the theme that changes. At puberty that theme is sexuality, love, partnership. The desire awakens for the opposite pole, for the 'you'. There is an urge to make contact with what the 'I' lacks – and yet at the same time a lack of confidence to do so. Sexual fantasies arise – only to lead in their turn to feelings of shame. It is truly enlightening, then, that such a conflict should make itself visible by way of the skin, for the skin is the boundary of the 'I' – that boundary that has to be transcended if the 'you' is ever to be discovered. At the same time the skin is the very organ via which we need to make contact in order to touch and caress. It is via our skin, similarly, that we need to please the other person if we are to receive their love.

In the presence of this 'red-hot' theme, then, the skin of pubescent youngsters becomes inflamed, thereby indicating not only that something is trying to burst through the former frontiers, some new energy itching to break out, but also that an attempt is being made to prevent it from breaking out, thanks to a fear of the newly awakened drive. Acne is a form of self-defence, in that it gets in the way of meeting people and so impedes sexual expression. The result is a vicious circle: the unexpressed sexuality shows up on the skin as acne, while the acne in turn gets in the way of sex. The repressed wish for sexual excitement turns into an excitation of the skin. The close link between sex and acne can be seen clearly from the sites where the latter occurs. Acne appears exclusively on the face and – in the case of girls – on the neckline, apart from occasionally affecting the back. The rest of the skin remains unaffected by acne, since it would serve no purpose there. And so youngsters' embarrassment about their sexuality is transposed into embarrassment about their spots.

For treating acne many doctors prescribe the Pill to good effect. The symbolism underlying this effect is readily apparent: the Pill feigns pregnancy in the body, thus at the same time mimicking what would have happened had sex already taken place – and so the acne disappears, because it has no further need to serve its preventive function. Sunbathing and seaside holidays usually reduce acne considerably, while it tends to get progressively worse the more the body is wrapped up. Certainly clothing's function as a 'second skin' emphasises delimitation and untouchability, whereas stripping off is already the first step towards self-opening, with the sun acting as a harmless replacement for the warmth of another body that the patient at once so longs for and so fears. And in the final event it is a well-known fact that a full experience of sex itself is the best treatment for acne.

Everything that we have said about acne at puberty applies in large measure to nearly all skin eruptions. Rashes always indicate that something which has hitherto been held back (repressed) is trying to break through the confines imposed by the repression in order to come to light (to consciousness). A rash allows something that was previously invisible to show itself. This makes it perfectly understandable that nearly all childhood diseases such as measles, scarlet fever and rubella (German measles) should express themselves via the skin. With every childhood illness something new is breaking through into the child's life, which is why every childhood illness generally brings with it a powerful stride forward in personal development. The greater the efflorescence, the more quickly the illness runs its course – the eruption succeeds, in other words. 'Milk crust' (impetigo) in infants may be seen as a response to mothers who touch their children too little or neglect them emotionally. The 'milk crust' is a visible expression of this invisible wall and an attempt to break through the resulting isolation. Eczema, meanwhile, is often used by mothers to justify their inner aversion to their children. The mothers concerned are for the most part particularly 'aesthetic' people who themselves attach great importance to keeping the skin clean.

One of the most common skin diseases is *psoriasis*. This manifests itself in clearly delineated discs or patches of inflamed tissue covered with silvery-white scales. In psoriasis the process by which the skin naturally forms a horny outer layer is exaggerated out of all proportion. One cannot help but be reminded of armour-plating (compare the horny armour of some animals). But in this case the skin's natural protective function has been turned into a form of armour: the sufferers in question are shutting themselves off in both directions. They are no longer willing to let anything either in or out. Reich's highly appropriate term for the effects of psychological defensiveness and walling oneself off was 'character armour'. Behind every form of defence there lies a fear of getting hurt. The greater our defensiveness and the thicker our armour, the greater are our inner sensitivity and our fear of injury.

Much the same happens in the animal kingdom. Take away the scales of a scaly animal, and inside we find a soft, unprotected, vulnerable thing. Those of us who are so defensive as to refuse to let anybody or anything in are usually the most sensitive. A hard shell often hides a soft kernel. Yet the attempt to protect a vulnerable soul with such armour is not without its tragic side. Granted that the armour shields us from being wounded or hurt; yet at the same time it also shields us from everything else too, including love and devotion. Love means opening ourselves up – yet that, too, is prejudiced by a defensive attitude. So it is that our armour hems us in, cutting our soul off from the land of the living – and in the process our fear starts to grow all the more. It becomes ever more difficult to break out of this vicious circle. At some point we have to allow to happen what we have all along been so afraid of and so determined to resist – we actually have to *let* the psyche get hurt, in order to learn that it is not in the slightest danger of going under as a result. We have to accept the *wounds* in order to experience the true *wonder*. This step occurs only under the external pressure that either our destiny or psychotherapy itself can bring to bear on us.

We have gone into the link between excessive vulnerability and self-armouring at this point in rather greater detail for the very good reason that psoriasis itself physically demonstrates the link in question very strikingly. Psoriasis, after all, leads to open places in the skin, to cracks and bleeding sores. This in turn places the skin at risk of infection. We can thus see how the extremes come into close conjunction with each other at this point, how the woundedness and the horny armour bring to light the conflict between the desire for intimacy on the one hand and the fear of intimacy on the other. Psoriasis often begins on the elbows. But then it is with the elbows that we 'elbow our way through': it is also with the elbows that we 'prop ourselves up'. And it is at precisely these points that hardening and vulnerability duly appear. In psoriasis, self-delimitation and isolation reach their extreme point, thus forcing the patient – physically, at least – to become 'open and vulnerable' once again.

Itching (Pruritus)

Itching is a phenomenon which accompanies many skin ailments (urticaria or nettle-rash, for example), but it can also occur by itself, without any particular 'cause'. Itching can drive us almost to distraction; we are constantly obliged to scratch some part of the body or other. Linguistically, the general idea of itching and scratching also has a purely psychological meaning: 'I'm itching to do it,' we say, or again, 'I was tickled pink.' Now itching and tickling are both forms of stimulation, and the verb 'to stimulate' covers a whole spectrum of experience ranging from simple charm, delight, fascination and attraction, through common-or-garden tickling, teasing, provocation and/or irritation, to outright excitement, thrill and arousal. While it is true that many of these words have possible sexual connotations, we should not let sheer sexuality blind us to all their other meanings and possible references – many of which may appear at first sight to be contradictory. We can 'irritate' people in an aggressive way, and yet at the same time we may describe the mood of a delightful evening as 'stimulating'. If something 'excites a fascination' for us, it arouses something in us – be it sexuality, aggression, affection or love. Thus, is it not possible to attach any single, clear valuation to the idea of stimulation. For us it is ambivalent. None of us can be certain whether we shall find any given stimulus delightful or be irritated by it. All that can be said is that a stimulus *stimulates us*. Even the Latin word *prurigo* means not only 'itching' but also 'lasciviousness' and 'lust', while the corresponding verb *prurire* means 'to itch'.

A physical itch shows that something is 'biting' us or 'bugging' us on the psychological level. Yet evidently we have ignored it or refused to notice it on that level, or else it would have had no need to somatise itself as an itch in the first place. Behind the itching stands some powerful emotion, some inner fire, some burning issue that wants to come out into the open and be discovered. That is why it itches and so makes us scratch. Scratching is a mild form of scraping and digging. Just as we scrape and dig the earth in order to find something buried and bring it to light, so pruritus patients scratch the surface of their skin in order symbolically to find what is bugging them, biting them, needling them or exciting them. Once they have found out what is making them so edgy they feel less itchy. And so itching always warns us of something that is 'biting us' or 'needling us'. It informs us of something that, far from 'leaving us cold', is 'burning us up inside': a glowing passion, a fiery enthusiasm, a burning love or even a flaming anger. No wonder, then, that itching so often goes with skin eruptions, red spots and *in-flamed* 'places'. The challenge is to keep scratching around in our consciousness until we have found what is really biting us. It promises to be a truly stimulating experience!

SKIN DISEASES

In the event of skin-problems and eruptions, the following are the questions to ask yourself:

1. Am I delimiting myself too much?
2. How easy am I finding it to make contact with other people?
3. Is there a repressed desire for intimacy behind my tendency to reject others?
4. What is it that is trying to burst through the barriers so as to come to light? (sexuality? instinctiveness? passion? aggression? enthusiasm?)
5. What is it that is really 'getting under my skin'?
6. Have I condemned myself to solitary confinement?

Eight

The Kidneys

Within the human body the kidneys represent the realm of partnership. Kidney pains and diseases always appear when we are engaged in conflicts with our partners. What is meant by 'partnership' here, though, is not just sexuality, but the fundamental way in which we approach our fellow human beings. Our particular approach to other people can be seen at its clearest within a partnership, but it applies just as much to anybody else with whom we come into contact. In order to gain a better understanding of the relationship between the kidneys and the general subject of partnership, it may be useful at this point to start by taking a look at the psychological background to any relationship.

The very polarity of our consciousness means that we are not aware of our own wholeness, but only ever identify ourselves with one particular aspect of our nature. This aspect we call the 'I'. The missing aspect is our shadow, and this, by definition, we are unaware of. Humanity's path is the path towards greater awareness. We are constantly forced to make conscious those aspects of the shadow of which we were previously unaware and to integrate them into our I-dentification. This learning process can only come to an end when we finally attain total consciousness – when, in a word, we are 'whole'. This oneness encompasses the whole of polarity within its undividedness, and not least masculinity and femininity.

The perfect human being is androgynous – in other words, has fused both his or her masculine and feminine aspects into a psychological unity (the so-called 'Alchemical Wedding'). Androgyny is not to be confused with hermaphrodism, however. Clearly, androgyny applies only on the psychological level: the body itself retains its gender. But the consciousness no longer identifies itself with it (rather as an infant also has a physical gender without identifying itself with it). The goal of androgyny finds its outward expression not only in celibacy, but also (in a man, at least) in the robes of a priest or monk. 'Being a man' implies identifying oneself with the masculine pole of the psyche, as a result of which the feminine aspect automatically slips into the shadows; 'being a woman', similarly, implies identifying oneself with the feminine psychological pole, as a result of which it is the masculine pole that is consigned to a shadow existence. It is our task to make ourselves aware of our shadow. But we can only do this via the medium of projection. We have to seek out and find what we are lacking via the outer world, even though it is really inside us all the time.

To start with, of course, this sounds paradoxical – and perhaps it is for that reason that it is so seldom understood. Yet all knowledge demands at its very outset the division of subject from object. The eye, for example, is perfectly capable of seeing, but has no hope of ever seeing *itself* – it can only do so via the medium of projection onto a reflecting surface. This is the only way in which we can ever know ourselves: as human beings we are in the self-same boat. A man can only become aware of the feminine aspect of his psyche (C. G. Jung called it the *anima*) by projecting it onto a physical woman. The same applies to a woman, but in reverse. We can imagine the shadow as being composed of layers. There are very deep layers which evoke dread in us, and of which we are therefore terrified; and there are other layers that lie closer to the surface, only waiting to be worked on and made conscious. If I now meet somebody who is living out for real some aspect which *in me* lies in this uppermost part of the shadow, I fall in love with that person. But the words 'that person' apply not merely to the actual human being 'out there', but also to the 'inner person' represented by the relevant aspect of my own shadow, for both are ultimately one and the same.

In the last resort, then, whatever it is that we like or hate about another person always lies within ourselves. We speak of 'love' when somebody else reflects an area of our own shadow that we are keen to get to know better; but we call it 'hate' when somebody reflects a very deep level of our shadow that we are at present totally unwilling to encounter inwardly. We find the other sex attractive because it represents something that we are lacking. Yet at the same time we are often afraid of it because it is a 'something' of which we are unconscious. The encounter with a partner is an encounter with the unknown aspect of our inner psyche. Once we are fully aware of this mechanism via which the various aspects of our shadows are reflected in others, we can start to see all our problems of relationship in a new light. All the difficulties that we have with our partners are in fact difficulties with ourselves.

Our relationship with our unconscious is always ambivalent – it excites us, and yet we are all afraid of it. Our relationships with our partners are normally just as ambivalent. We love them *and* hate them; we are determined to possess them totally *and* intent on getting rid of them; we find them wonderful *and* dreadful. In all the activities and squabbles that go to make up a relationship, we are always working on our own shadows. That is why contrary types so often come together. *Opposites attract each other*, as everybody knows, and yet people persist in wondering aloud 'why those two ever came together, seeing that they are so incompatible'. In fact, however, the greater the contrast, the more suited they actually are, for each lives out the other's shadow or – more to the point – each leaves the other to do that living out for him or her instead. Partnerships between two very similar people are admittedly less risky and more cosy, but by and large they contribute very little to the development of either party; it is only the participants' own, conscious aspects that get reflected in each other – a situation that is ultimately both bland and boring. Both parties find each other 'wonderful' and project their common shadow onto the rest of the world around them, which they then do their common utmost to avoid. It is only the friction in a relationship that is fruitful, for it is only by working on our shadow in and through the other person that we eventually come closer to ourselves. At which point it should become obvious that the goal of this work is nothing less than *our own wholeness*.

Ideally, the end of a partnership should see two individuals who have both become whole in themselves, or who at least – if we are to be less idealistic – have become *more* whole as a result of illuminating the unconscious aspects of their own souls and integrating them into their respective consciousnesses. That end is not fulfilled by the typical pair of cooing doves who insist that they 'cannot live without each other'. Such assertions merely reveal that those involved are, out of sheer convenience (one could say cowardice), merely using each other to live out their shadows for them, without making any attempt to work on their own projections or take them back again onto their own shoulders. In such cases (and they are the vast majority!) neither partner allows the other to develop any further because this would throw into question their established roles. If either subsequently undergoes psychotherapy, the partner quite often complains about the changes that have occurred . . . ('But we only wanted the symptom to go away!')

A partnership has only attained its goal when neither needs the other any more. Only in this event has the promise of 'eternal love' actually been taken seriously. Love is an act of consciousness that involves opening up the frontiers of our awareness to the object of our love with a view to total union. But this has only happened if we have absorbed into our soul everything that the partner represents or (to put it another way) if we have withdrawn our projections and reunited ourselves with them. At which point the other person has become free of his or her role as a projection-screen – free either of attraction or of repulsion for us – and so love has become eternal (that is, independent of time) since it has become realised within our own soul. Such considerations, though, always tend to frighten people who are firmly bound by their projections to the physical world. They attach their love to the formal manifestation, rather than to the psychological content. With such an attitude, the impermanence of earthly things becomes a threat, whereupon those involved live in hopes of meeting their 'loved ones' again in the Beyond. But this is to overlook the fact that the 'Beyond' is actually here all the time. The Beyond is simply the realm that lies beyond the world of forms. Everything visible is merely a metaphor: why should things be any different where people are concerned?

Our life's aim is to make the visible world superfluous – and that goes for our partner too. Problems only arise when two people 'use' their relationship in different ways – with the one working on his or her projections and reabsorbing them again, while the other remains firmly stuck in the world of projection. This eventually leads to the point when the one becomes independent of the other, while the other's heart is fit to break. If, on the other hand, both parties remain stuck with their projections, we have a case of love 'till death do us part' – and thereafter great grief because the other half isn't there any more. Happy are those who grasp the fact that the only thing that cannot be taken from them is what they have realised in themselves. Love's aim is nothing if not oneness. All the while it is still directed towards external objects it has not yet attained its goal.

It is important for us to understand clearly the inner structure of a partnership if we are to follow the analogical relationship between it and what goes on in the kidneys. We find in the body both single organs (such as the stomach, the liver, the pancreas and the spleen) and organs arranged in pairs (such as the lungs, the testicles, the ovaries and the kidneys). If we consider the paired organs, it is noticeable that they all have some link with the themes of contact and partnership. Thus, the lungs represent the sphere of informal contact and communication whereas, as genital organs, the testicles and ovaries represent sexuality. At the same time the kidneys correspond to partnership, to intimate human relationships. Moreover, these three areas also correspond to the three ancient Greek terms for love – *philia* (friendship), *eros* (sexual love) and *agape* (gradual self-unification with all things).

All the substances that are absorbed by the body eventually finish up in the blood. It is the kidneys' job to act as a central filtration plant. For this they need to be able to recognise which substances are beneficial to the organism and can be put to good use, and which are waste products and toxins that need to be excreted. For this onerous task the kidneys have at their disposal various mechanisms, which in the light of their physiological complexity we propose to simplify here into two basic functions. The first stage of the filtering process works along the lines of a mechanical sieve, with particles above a certain size being retained. The pores of this sieve are of exactly the right size to hold back the smallest protein-molecule (albumen). The second, much more complicated stage is based on a mixture of osmosis and the contraflow principle. In its essentials, osmosis is based on a balancing act between the pressures and concentrations of two fluids on either side of a semi-permeable membrane. In the process the contraflow principle sees to it that these two different, concentrated fluids are repeatedly passed next to each other, with the result that if necessary the kidneys can excrete highly concentrated urine (morning urine, for example). It is the ultimate aim of this osmotic balancing act to ensure that the body is able to retain the vital salts on which (among other things) the acid/alkaline balance depends.

The layman is for the most part totally unaware of the literally vital importance to us of this acid/alkaline balance, which is expressed numerically in terms of pH values. Thus, all biochemical reactions (energy-production and protein-synthesis, for example) depend to within very narrow limits on the preservation of a given pH value. The blood, in particular, maintains a level at the exact mid-point between alkaline and acid, between yin and yang. In the same way, every partnership amounts to an attempt to bring both poles – both masculine (yang, acid) and feminine (yin, alkaline) – into harmonious equilibrium. Just as the kidneys see to it that the balance between acid and alkaline is guaranteed, so a partnership similarly sees to it that we work towards fulfilling our wholeness through a relationship whereby another person lives out our shadow for us. In this way the 'other' (or 'better') 'half' makes up via his or her very essence for whatever we ourselves are lacking.

The biggest danger in any relationship, meanwhile, is the conviction that all problematic or disturbing forms of behaviour are the other person's 'pigeon' and have nothing to do with us. In such cases we are simply getting bogged down in our own projections and failing to recognise the necessity and value of working on our own shadow area – as reflected in our partner – as a means of becoming more aware and so of contributing to our own growth and maturation. Should this error manifest itself in bodily form, the kidneys go on to allow vital substances such as proteins and salts to pass through its filter-systems, thus losing to the environment components that are important for the body's own development (as in the case of glomerulonephritis, for example). In the process the kidneys show the self-same inability to recognise their own in the matter of vital substances as the psyche does in refusing to recognise its own in the matter of important problems and in consequently leaving it all to the other person. Just as we each need to recognise ourselves in our partners, so the kidneys similarly need to be able to recognise those 'foreign' substances from outside that are vital for getting to grips with things and so developing further. Just how strong a link there is between the kidneys and the subject of partnership and sociability is something that can also be seen quite easily from certain customs of everyday life. On almost every occasion when people get together to establish contacts, drinking plays a vital part. And no wonder, for drinking stimulates the 'contact organs' that are the kidneys, and thus also our ability to make contact. The moment we start clinking our brimming glasses and beer-mugs together, that contact soon becomes closer still. Via the medium of the glass-clinking we can happily flirt with each other without giving offence. Even the change from polite, distant forms of address to their more familiar, 'chummy' counterparts is nearly always linked with some kind of drinking ritual, with the drink acting as a kind of libation to fraternisation. In fact any establishment of human contact without some kind of communal drinking is all but inconceivable. Whether at a party, a social get-together or a folk-festival, people universally use drink to give them the 'Dutch courage' to make approaches to each other. All the more suspiciously, then, do such circles regard those who decline to join in the drinking; for those who drink nothing (or little) are showing that they do not want to excite their contact organs – that they wish to keep their distance. On such occasions, meanwhile, people distinctly prefer strongly diuretic drinks that stimulate the kidneys particularly sharply, such as coffee, tea and alcohol. (Straight after the social drinking, moreover, comes the equally significant activity of smoking. Smoking stimulates those other contact-organs of ours that are the lungs. It is common knowledge that people generally smoke far more in company than they do when they are alone.) Those of us who drink a lot are showing that they want contact; but their danger lies in getting stuck on the level of substitute gratifications.

Kidney stones occur as the result of the deposition and crystallisation of certain substances that are present in the urine in excessive quantities (for example uric acid, calcium phosphate and calcium oxalate). In addition to the various environmental conditions that are responsible, the risk of stone-formation correlates strongly with the amount of liquid drunk; large quantities of liquid lower the concentration of these substances and raise their solubility. If a stone nevertheless forms, this interrupts the flow and can lead to an attack of colic. Colic is a perfectly sensible attempt on the part of the body to expel the stony obstruction through peristaltic movements of the ureter. This extremely painful process can be compared to a birth. The colic pain leads to extreme agitation and a strong urge to squirm about. Indeed, if the body's own colic fails to shift the stone, doctors themselves ask patients to jump around on their own account in a further attempt to get the stone moving again. In addition, the treatment attempts to hasten the 'birth' of the stone mainly through relaxation, warm applications and plenty of fluids.

The correspondences on the psychological level are easy to see. The obstructing stone consists of substances that in fact ought to have been excreted, since they have nothing more to contribute to the body's development. The stone thus corresponds to a whole host of themes of which the patient ought long since to have let go in the light of their inapplicability to his or her further development. 'Hanging on regardless' to unimportant themes – to 'water' that should long since have been allowed to flow 'under the bridge' – merely obstructs the flow and produces a blockage. The symptomatology of colic then forces the very movement that the patient was so keen to prevent by hanging on, and the doctor demands of the patient exactly the right thing – that he or she should jump around.

Only a leap out of the old can set our development in motion again and free us from all our superannuated clutter (the stone).

Statistics reveal that men suffer more frequently from kidney stones than women. The themes of harmony and partnership are more difficult for men to come to terms with than for women, who are by nature more in tune with such principles. For women, by contrast, aggressive self-assertion is a bigger problem, for this is a principle that comes more naturally to men. (This shows up statistically in the already mentioned higher frequency of *gall*stones in women.) The therapeutic measures applied to kidney colic meanwhile outline particularly well the principles that are useful in solving problems of harmony and relationship: warmth as an expression of devotion and love, relaxation of the constricted channels as signs of self-opening and self-broadening, and finally the administration of liquids to bring everything back into motion and flux again.

Fibrosis of the Kidney and the Artificial Kidney

The end of the road is reached when all the kidneys' functions finally pack up totally and a machine – the artificial kidney – has to take over the vital tasks of blood-purification. At this point it is the 'perfect machine' that takes over the role of partner, in the light of patients' unreadiness to use living partners to get to grips with their problems. If no partner has proved sufficiently perfect or dependable, or the desire for freedom and independence has proved too overwhelming, patients go on to find in the artificial kidney a partner that is both ideal and perfect, in that it does everything asked of it faithfully and dependably without making any personal demands or imposing its own needs. By the same token, though, patients are also totally dependent on it. At least three times a week they have to rendezvous with it in hospital or – in the event that they can afford a machine of their own – must sleep night after night faithfully by its side. They can never stray far from it, and possibly learn in this way that there is really no such thing as a perfect partner – so long as we are still not complete in ourselves, that is.

KIDNEY DISEASE

If something is 'going to your kidneys', address yourself to the following questions:

1. What problems am I having in the area of my current partnership?
2. Do I have a tendency to get stuck with my own projections, and thus to regard my partner's problems as his or hers alone?
3. Am I neglecting to recognise myself in all my partner's quirks of behaviour?
4. Am I clinging on to old problems and so stopping the flow of my own further development?
5. What forward leap is my kidney stone really trying to encourage me to take?

The Bladder

The bladder is the reservoir in which all the substances excreted by the kidneys as urine await their opportunity to leave the body. The pressure caused by the sheer bulk of urine eventually forces us to release it, and this leads to a feeling of relief. But we all know from experience that the urge to urinate is also very often linked conspicuously to certain types of situation. These are always situations in which we are being put under psychological pressure – whether they be examinations, therapy or whatever – involving anticipatory fears or stress-related conditions. The pressure which is initially experienced psychologically is shifted down into the bladder and here experienced in the form of actual physical pressure.

Pressure always demands of us that we let go and relax. If this fails to occur at the psychological level, we are obliged to allow it to happen physically via the bladder. In this way it becomes patently obvious to us how great the pressure of any given situation really is, how painful it is likely to become if we fail to let go of it, and how liberating, by contrast, that letting-go can be. Furthermore, this particular form of somatisation also permits us to transform whatever pressure we are currently experiencing passively into active pressure, in that we can interrupt and manipulate almost any situation by insisting that we 'have to go to the toilet'. Anybody who has to go to the toilet is aware of being under pressure, but at the same time is *exercising* pressure, too – as every schoolchild ('first-year bladder') and every patient knows: he or she therefore invariably uses this particular symptom with unerring accuracy, if at the same time generally unconsciously.

The link between symptom and power-ploy – a link which is particularly obvious in this case – also plays a not inconsiderable role in all our other symptoms, too. Every patient tends to use his or her symptoms as levers of power. And with this we are touching on one of the strongest taboos of our time. The exercise of power is one of humanity's most fundamental problems. So long as we have an 'I', we strive to dominate and to extend our power. Every '. . . but *I* want' is an expression of this quest for ego-dominance. But since power has become a concept that is nowadays very much tinged with negativity, people see themselves as forced to cloak their various power-ploys in ever better disguises. Relatively few people have the courage to declare openly their will to power or to live it out honestly. The majority of us attempt to fulfil our repressed power-urges indirectly. For this we above all exploit such areas as illness and social disadvantage. These areas are relatively safe from disclosure, in view of the fact that projecting all blame onto mechanical processes and the rest of the world around us is nowadays universally regarded as perfectly acceptable and legitimate.

Since virtually all of us use more or less these same areas for our power-strategies, nobody is interested in taking the lid off what is going on – indeed, any attempt to do so is met with the deepest indignation. Illness and death are regularly used to submit the world to extortion. By being ill we can nearly always achieve things that we could never have got in the absence of symptoms – devotion, sympathy, money, time off, help and/or control over others. This secondary advantage of illness – the fact that symptoms can be used as instruments of power – quite often gets in the way of healing.

Returning to our current topic, then, it is quite easy to detect the theme of 'symptoms as expressions of power' in the particular case of bed-wetting. If a child spends all day under such strong pressures (whether from parents or from school) that it can neither let go nor express its own needs, nocturnal bed-wetting solves several problems at once: it provides the chance to let go in response to the pressures being experienced, and at the same time it offers the child the opportunity to condemn its otherwise all-powerful parents to utter helplessness. By way of this particular symptom, in fact, the child is able to return in safely disguised form all the pressure that it is put under during the day. At the same time we should not overlook the link between bed-wetting and crying. Both of them serve to unload and release inner pressures by way of 'letting go'. We could thus describe bed-wetting as a kind of 'lower-level crying'.

The themes that we have just been discussing are relevant to all the remaining bladder conditions too. When the bladder is inflamed, the burning sensation experienced while passing water shows very clearly how painful the patient finds it to let go. A frequent urge to urinate, with little or no urine actually being passed, is an expression of a total inability to let go despite all the pressures. And with none of these symptoms should it ever be forgotten that the substances (and, psychologically, the themes) involved have all outlived their usefulness and now only represent so much excess baggage.

BLADDER CONDITIONS

Bladder problems throw up the following questions:

1. What areas am I clinging on to despite the fact that they have long since outlived their usefulness and are only waiting to be got rid of?
2. Where am I putting myself under pressure and then projecting that pressure onto others (examinations, the boss)?
3. Which well-worn theme is it time for me to let go of?
4. What have I got to cry about?

Nine

Sexuality and Pregnancy

Sexuality is the sphere in which human beings most commonly get to practical grips with the theme of polarity. It is here that we are each made aware of our incompleteness and therefore set out to seek what we are lacking. We unite ourselves physically with our antipole, and in that union experience a new state of consciousness that we call 'orgasm'. We perceive this state of consciousness as the quintessence of bliss. It has only one disadvantage: it cannot be prolonged in time. Generally people attempt to offset this disadvantage by sheer frequency of repetition. Brief though the moment of bliss may be each time, it nevertheless shows us that there are states of being available to our consciousness that are qualitatively far superior to our 'normal' consciousness. In the last event it is precisely this feeling of bliss that never lets us rest, that turns us into eternal seekers. For sexuality at least reveals the first half of the secret: if we unite two polarities so that they become one, ecstasy is spread abroad. Ecstasy is consequently a state of union. All that we are lacking is that second half of the secret which will show us how we can remain in this state of consciousness, in this ecstasy, for good, without ever declining from it again. The answer is simple: all the while the union of opposites is achieved only on the physical level (sexuality), the resulting state of consciousness (orgasm) is also temporally circumscribed, since the law of time underlies all physical existence. We can become free of time only by bringing about the union of opposites in our consciousness as well: once I have achieved union on this level, I have attained eternal (that is, timeless) ecstasy of soul.

It is with this realisation that the esoteric path begins which in the East is also called the path of yoga. 'Yoga' is a Sanskrit word meaning 'yoke' (compare the Latin word *jugum*, which also means 'yoke'). A yoke always combines a duality into a unity – two oxen, two buckets, or whatever. Yoga is the art of uniting dualities. Since sexuality contains within itself the fundamental paradigm of this path, while at the same time representing it on a level that is accessible to everybody, sexuality has in all epochs been freely used as an analogical representation of this self-same path. Even today, baffled tourists continue to be astonished at what they take to be the pornographic images displayed on oriental temples. Yet here the sexual union of two divine figures is simply being used to represent symbolically the great secret of *conjunctio oppositorum*, or the union of opposites.

It is one of the peculiarities of Christian theology that over the course of its development it took to denigrating the body, and sexuality in particular, to such an extent that as children we were taught to see sex and the 'spiritual path' as great irreconcilable opposites (naturally sexual symbolism was not always alien to Christians, as the example of the doctrine of the 'bride of Christ' clearly shows). In so many groups that regard themselves as 'esoteric' this conceptual opposition of flesh to spirit is still carefully cultivated. In such circles there is a fundamental confusion between transmuting and repressing. Even here, though, it should suffice to understand the esoteric axiom 'as Above, so Below'. It follows from this, after all, that whatever we cannot cope with at the lower level we certainly cannot cope with at the higher level. Those of us who have sexual problems should thus take steps to solve them on the physical level, not seek salvation in flight – for on the 'higher' level uniting the opposites is much more difficult still!

Seen from this angle, it is perhaps understandable why Freud should have reduced virtually all human problems to questions of sexuality. This step was thoroughly justified in its way, except that it had just one small formal defect. Freud (and all those who think along the same lines) neglected to take the final step from the level of concrete manifestation to the principle which underlies it. Sexuality is in fact only *one* of the possible manifestations of the principle of polarity or the union of opposites. At this abstract level even Freud's critics could no doubt agree: all human problems can be reduced to the question of polarity and our attempts to unite the opposites (it was C. G. Jung who eventually undertook this final step). Nevertheless it is certainly correct that most of us first learn of, experience and concern ourselves with the problems of polarity on the sexual level, which is why sexuality and partnership provide the raw materials for most of our conflicts. It is here that the theme of polarity makes things so difficult for us as to drive us to *distraction*, until we eventually discover for ourselves that ultimate point of unity.

Menstrual Problems

A woman's monthly periods are an expression of femininity, fertility and receptivity. She is totally at the mercy of this rhythm. For all the restrictions that it places on her, she has no choice but to comply with it. With this compliance we touch on one of the central aspects of femininity – namely the faculty of self-surrender. In speaking here of 'femininity', we are of course referring to the general principle of the feminine pole of existence – as referred to by the Chinese, for example, as 'yin', as symbolised by the alchemists in terms of the moon, or as expressed by depth psychology via the symbolism of water. Each individual woman is from this viewpoint merely one particular concrete manifestation of the archetypal feminine. The feminine principle can best be defined in terms of receptivity. As the *I Ching* puts it, 'The way of the creative brings about the masculine, the way of the receptive brings about the feminine.' And, at another point, 'The receptive is the most self-sacrificial in the world.'

The faculty of self-surrender is the feminine's central quality: it is the basis of all the other feminine qualities, such as openness, receptivity, sensitivity and protectiveness. At the same time, self-surrender implies a renunciation of positive action. Consider, for example, those archetypal symbols of femininity: water and the moon. Both of them eschew all active radiation or emission on their own account, unlike their opposites, fire and the sun. As a result they become capable of receiving, absorbing and reflecting light and warmth. Water renounces all claim to shape or form, instead taking on any form presented to it. It adapts, surrenders itself.

Behind the polarities of sun and moon, fire and water, masculine and feminine there is, however, no value-judgement. In fact any such valuation would be absolutely pointless, since both poles in isolation are un-whole, mere half-entities, with each needing the other pole for its own completion. Yet this completeness is attainable only if both poles fully manifest their specific individualities. In many arguments about emancipation this archetypal law is too easily overlooked. It would be crass stupidity for water to complain that it cannot burn or shine, and to deduce from this that it is somehow inferior. Neither pole is any better or worse than the other; they are merely different. It is from this very polar differentiatedness, indeed, that the tension arises which we call 'life'. The union of opposites is not to be attained by blurring the differences between the poles. A woman who fully accepts and lives out her own femininity will never feel herself to be in any way 'inferior'.

It is a failure to reconcile oneself to one's own femininity that is nevertheless the basis of most menstrual problems, as well as of a good many other symptoms in the sexual sphere. Self-surrender and being prepared to go along with things is always a difficult challenge for us to face, given that it demands a renunciation of 'I will', a renunciation of ego-dominance. We each have to give up something of our ego, sacrifice a part of ourselves, surrender a part of ourselves – just as the woman's monthly period itself demands. For with her blood the woman sacrifices something of her own life-force. Menstruation is both a 'little pregnancy' and a 'little birth'. To the extent that a woman is not prepared to be 'bound' in this way, menstrual problems or disturbances duly arise. They point to the fact that some (often unconscious) determinant within the woman is refusing to give in, whether to menstruation itself, to sex or to the male partner. It is precisely to this rebellious 'But I don't want to' that advertisements for sanitary towels and tampons deliberately appeal. They promise women that using the product in question will make them independent, enabling them to do whatever they like regardless of the day of the month. In this way the advertisements home in on the woman's actual point of conflict: 'Be a woman, certainly – but don't go along with everything that being a woman brings with it.'

Those who have painful periods are in fact finding it painful to be a woman. From menstrual problems, consequently, we can deduce that there are also sexual problems, for the protest against self-surrender that shows up in menstrual problems also gets in the way of letting go in the context of one's sex-life. Those who can let go in orgasm are also capable of letting go in the menstrual context. Orgasm, like going to sleep, is a kind of 'little death'. Menstruation is also a process involving a 'little death', for in the process tissues die off and are expelled. But dying is nothing less than a challenge to let go of our grasping egotism and our power games, and simply to let be. Death only ever threatens the ego, never the person as a whole. For those of us who cling on to our ego, death is a struggle. Orgasm is a 'little death' because it similarly demands that we let go of our 'I'. For orgasm is truly the union of *I* and *you*, and this presupposes an opening-up of the frontiers of the 'I'. Consequently those of us who hang on to the 'I' are denied orgasm (the same goes for going to sleep, as we shall see in a later chapter). What death, orgasm and menstruation have in common should thus be evident: it is our capacity for self-surrender, our willingness to sacrifice part of our ego.

In the light of this it is understandable why (as we saw earlier) anorexics for the most part either have no periods at all or have severe menstrual problems: their repressed urge to dominate is far too great for them to go along with it all. They are afraid of their own femininity, afraid of sexuality, fertility and motherhood. It is well-known that in situations of great fear and uncertainty, in catastrophes, prisons, work-camps and concentration camps women's periods often cease entirely (secondary amenorrhoea). All these situations are by their very nature unpropitious for self-surrender, but instead challenge the women concerned to start 'being their own men' and to become active and self-assertive.

There is a further menstrual connection that we ought not to overlook: menstruation is an expression of a woman's ability to have children. The onset of the monthly period has very different emotional effects according to whether the woman concerned wants a child or not. If she wants a child, the onset of the period is a sign for her that 'it hasn't worked again'. In such cases the prime symptom is a feeling of unwellness and a generally bad temper before and during the period. The bleeding is sensed as being a painful experience. Such women also prefer unsafe contraceptive techniques – this being a compromise between the unconscious desire for children and an actual alibi. If, on the other hand, the woman in question is afraid of having a child, she longs for the period to come – which can of course lead directly to its being delayed. Frequently what then ensues is a very long period of bleeding, which under certain circumstances can also be used as an excuse for avoiding sex. At bottom, after all, menstruation can – like any symptom – be used as an instrument of power, whether in order to prevent sex or to gain attention and tenderness.

Menstruation is controlled in the body by the combined influence of the female hormone oestrogen and the ovarian hormone progesterone. This mutual combination corresponds on the hormonal level to the duality of sexuality itself. If this balance is disturbed, the periods, too, are disturbed. It is very difficult to cure disturbances of this kind through the medical administration of hormones, for the hormones are merely physical representatives of the masculine and feminine aspects of the psyche. Healing can be achieved only by reconciling ourselves to our own sexual role, for this is the precondition for our subsequently being able to realise within ourselves the opposite sexual pole.

False Pregnancy (Pseudogravidity)

We can observe the somatising of psychological processes in particularly dramatic form in the case of imaginary pregnancy. It is not merely a question of subjective pregnancy symptoms such as food-cravings, feelings of fullness, nausea and vomiting; the women concerned go as far as to manifest the typical enlargement of the breasts, the pigmentation of the nipples and even the secretion of milk. They can feel the 'child' moving: their bodies swell up just like that of a heavily pregnant woman. The background to this phenomenon of false pregnancy – a relatively rare occurrence which has nevertheless been known about ever since antiquity – is the conflict between an extremely strong desire for children and an unconscious fear of responsibility. If false pregnancy appears in single women living in isolation, it can also point to a conflict between sexuality and motherhood. There is a desire to fulfil the 'noble' maternal role, without at the same time allowing 'ignoble' sex to play any part in it. In every version of false pregnancy, in fact, the body once again reveals the truth: it puffs itself up ... and all for nothing of any substance.

Problems in Pregnancy

Problems during pregnancy can reveal on some level, a degree of rejection of the child by the mother. Such an assertion will inevitably be repudiated most vehemently by those to whom it most closely applies. Yet if we are keen to discover the truth, if we really want to get to know ourselves, then we first of all have to let go of our habitual system of values. It is those values above all that get in the way of our being honest with ourselves. All the while we are convinced that we only have to adopt a given attitude or form of behaviour to become 'good people', we shall necessarily repress all those impulses which do not fit in with this scheme of things. It is these repressed impulses which then bring our nature back into its true balance by way of bodily symptoms.

This relationship needs to be stressed once again at this point, lest we deceive ourselves with an over-hasty response of 'But it just doesn't apply in my case!' Having children belongs directly to those themes that are most strongly hedged about with value-judgements, which is why so much dishonesty is transformed into actual symptoms in this particular area. Thus, any deficiency in this sphere shows that the woman in question wants to get rid of the child again – it is an unconscious abortion. In milder form, rejection of the child shows up in the (almost obligatory) nausea and above all in morning sickness. This symptom appears especially frequently in very slight, slender women, for pregnancy brings about within them a powerful surge of female hormone (oestrogen). It is precisely in women whose female self-identification is minimal, in other words, that this (hormonal) invasion of femininity releases the fear and resistance that shows up in nausea and vomiting. The general frequency of unwellness and nausea in pregnancy merely shows how commonly the expectation of a child leads not only to joy, but also to rejection. This is quite understandable in the light of the fact that having a child means a major upheaval in one's normal life and the adoption of responsibilities which may well fill one with fear initially. To the degree that we nevertheless fail to work on this sphere of conflict, our rejection is precipitated into the body.

Toxaemia

A distinction is normally drawn between early toxaemia (6 to 14 weeks) and the more serious late toxaemia. Toxaemia produces high blood-pressure, loss of protein via the kidneys, cramps (pre-eclampsia), nausea and morning-sickness. The overall picture reveals a resistance to the child, together with various part-physical, part-symbolic efforts to get rid of it. The protein that is excreted via the kidneys would actually have been of great value to the child itself. By losing it, however, one is seeing that it does not reach the child – endeavouring, in other words, to prevent the latter from growing by excreting the raw materials it needs. The cramps correspond to an attempt to expel the child (as in labour itself). All these relatively common symptoms reveal the conflict already described above. From the strength and dangerousness of the symptoms we can quite easily gauge how strongly accentuated the rejection of the child is or, by contrast, how far the mother is managing to work toward acknowledging her child.

In late toxaemia, though, we are at once faced with a much more extreme picture which puts not just the baby, but the mother too, at grave risk. With this condition the blood-flow through the placenta is severely restricted. The exchange-surface within the placenta measures twelve to fourteen square metres in area. With toxaemia this area is reduced to some seven square metres, and at four-and-a-half square metres the foetus dies. The placenta is the contact-surface between mother and child. If the blood-flow through it is throttled, the life-component is withdrawn from this contact. Thus it is that placental deficiency leads in a third of all cases to the death of the child. If an infant survives late toxaemia, it is generally very small and under-nourished, and looks just like an old person. Late toxaemia is an attempt on the part of the body to throttle the child, in the process of which the mother herself risks her own life.

Medically, those at risk from toxaemia are reckoned to include female diabetics, kidney patients and very overweight women. If we contemplate all three of these groups from our own point of view, it becomes clear that they all have a common problem – namely love. Diabetics cannot accept love and there-fore can give none either; kidney patients have partnership problems; and overweight patients reveal through their craving for food that they are attempting to compensate for their lack of love with food. Consequently it is not very surprising that women who have problems with love should also have difficul-ties in being open to childbearing.

Childbirth and Nursing

All problems that delay childbirth or make it difficult are ultimately signs of an attempt to hang on to the child and a refusal to give it up. This age-old problem between mother and child is later on repeated all over again when the child wants to leave the parental home. It is merely the self-same situation repeated on two different levels: at birth the child leaves the protection of the womb, and later on it leaves the protection of the parental home. Both cases lead to a 'difficult birth', until eventually the cord is successfully severed. Once again, then, the name of the subject at issue is 'letting go'.

The more deeply we penetrate into human symptomatology, and thus into human problems, the clearer it becomes that the whole of human life hovers between the two poles of 'letting in' and 'letting go'. The first of these we often also call 'love', the second – in its ultimate form – 'death'. Living involves practising letting in and letting go rhythmically. Often we can do only one and not the other: sometimes we can do neither. In the course of sex the woman has already been challenged to open herself up and enlarge herself in order to let in the *other*. Now, with childbirth, she is being challenged all over again to open herself up and enlarge herself, but this time so as to let go of a part of her own being in order that it may itself turn into the *other*.

Should she fail in this, birth complications or a caesarean section ensue. Overdue babies are frequently dragged into the light of day by means of a caesarean section, with the overdueness being in this case the mother's way of expressing her unwillingness to part company. The other grounds for a caesarean operation are likewise expressions of the same problem: the women concerned are afraid of being 'too tight', of a perineal rupture, or of being unattractive to their male partner.

It is the opposite problem, however, that we find in the case of premature childbirth, which is frequently brought on by a premature breaking of the uterine waters. This in turn is generally caused by premature labour and straining. It is an attempt to 'kick the child out'.

When a mother suckles her child, what happens is a good deal more than mere feeding. For the mother's milk contains antibodies which protect the child for the first six months. If the child receives no mother's milk, it also fails to receive this protection – and this in a sense that is a good deal more all-embracing than the matter of mere antibodies. If the child is not suckled, it lacks skin-contact with its mother: there is a lack of that protectiveness which is conveyed by the pressing of body against body. If an infant is not suckled, this shows that the mother is unwilling to feed and protect it, to intervene personally on behalf of the child. In mothers who cannot give milk this problem is a good deal more deeply repressed than in those who simply do not want to feed their children and are quite open about the fact.

Sterility (Inability to Conceive)

If a woman fails to have a child despite wanting one, this shows either that some unconscious resistance is present, or that her desire for a child is dishonestly motivated. An example of such a dishonest motivation is the hope of using the child to hang on to the partner or to force existing problems of relationship into the background. In such cases the body often reacts much more honestly and far-sightedly. In the same way, male impotence reveals a fear of the obligation and responsibility that having a child would bring with it.

The Menopause and Change of Life (Midlife Crisis)

Just like its original inception, the loss of menstruation comes across to a woman as a drastic change in her life. To her the menopause signals the loss of her fertility and at the same time the loss of a specifically female way of expressing herself. Just how this break in her life is taken and responded to by any given woman depends on her attitude to her own femininity thus far, and on how sexually fulfilled her life has been to date. Alongside the accompanying emotional reactions such as anxiety, irritability and loss of drive, which are all expressions of the fact that the entry into a new phase of life is being treated as a crisis, a further range of physical symptoms may be observed. Well-known among these are the so-called 'hot flushes' or 'hot flashes'. They are an attempt to demonstrate that the loss of menstruation does not necessarily mean any loss of womanhood in the sexual sense – to show that one is still 'in heat' and even 'a bit of hot stuff'. Renewed frequent bleeding similarly represents an attempt to feign continued fertility and youth.

Just how great the problems and complaints of the change of life turn out to be in practice depends to a large extent on how far the woman in question has succeeded in fulfilling her femininity to date. If she has not done so, all her unfulfilled desires pile up during this phase in the form of fears of being neglected, and lead to panic and attempts to 'catch up with the backlog'. It is only what we have not experienced that makes us 'hot'. It is generally during this phase, too, that benign tumours (known as myomas) frequently appear in the muscles of the uterus. These growths in the womb symbolise pregnancy: the women concerned cause something to grow in the womb that then has to be removed by an operation, just as though it were an actual delivery. Myoma should be taken as a cue for unearthing any lingering, unconscious desires to become pregnant.

Frigidity (Anorgasmia) and Impotence

Behind all sexual difficulties there stands fear. We have already spoken of the relationship between orgasm and death. Orgasm threatens our 'I', in that it releases a power which we can no longer direct or control with our ego. All ecstatic and rapturous conditions – no matter whether they be sexual or religious in nature – arouse in us both a delighted fascination and great fear at one and the same time. Fear predominates to the extent that we are used to controlling ourselves. Ecstasy is loss of control.

In our current society self-control is regarded as a highly positive quality, and we therefore take great pains to teach it to our children ('. . . now pull yourself together!'). This faculty of strict self-control makes it a good deal easier for us to live together socially, but at the same time is an expression of our society's amazing untruthfulness. Self-control means nothing less than repressing into the unconscious all those impulses that are unwelcome in society. As a result, the impulse duly disappears from sight, yet the question remains as to what happens to that impulse once it has been cleared out of the way. Since it is in the nature of an impulse to realise itself, it is bound to force itself back into visibility somehow, and consequently we have constantly to invest more energy in pushing the repressed impulse back underground and controlling it again.

At this point, then, it becomes clear why we are so afraid of losing control. An ecstatic or rapturous experience takes, as it were, the lid off the unconscious and allows everything that has hitherto been so carefully repressed to come to light once more. At which point we become honest to a degree, in that for the most part it turns out to be a pretty painful experience for us. *In vino veritas* – 'In the wine lies truth': this was something already known to the ancient Romans. Under the influence of drink even the gentlest lamb can become wildly aggressive, while 'hard-headed types' can break down in tears. The situation becomes truly honest, but socially more than a little disquieting – 'which is why people should be able to control themselves.' In which case it is then the hospital that eventually makes us honest.

If we are afraid of losing control and therefore make a daily habit of keeping a firm hold on ourselves, it is often extremely difficult suddenly to give up this ego-based control solely in the sexual context and to let things happen here of their own accord. In orgasm the 'little I' of which we are always so proud is simply blown away. In orgasm the 'I' dies (. . . unfortunately only temporarily, or enlightenment would be a much simpler matter!). But if we hold on to the 'I', we get in the way of orgasm. The more the 'I' keeps trying to make orgasm happen by sheer act of will, the less the prospect of success. Despite its familiarity, the full implications of this law are not generally appreciated. All the while the 'I' wants something, it is not to be attained. The desire of the ego ultimately turns into its opposite: *trying* to go to sleep merely keeps us awake; *wanting* to be potent leads to impotence. All the while the 'I' wants to become enlightened, the goal remains for ever out of reach! Orgasm is the renunciation of the 'I', yet only 'becoming one' can make this possible, for all the while an 'I' still exists, there is also a 'not-I', and so we are still subject to duality. Letting go and letting be is something that is demanded of both men and women alike if they are to achieve orgasm. Yet alongside this common theme men and women also need to realise quite different themes specific to their own particular sex if the upshot is to be a harmonious sexuality.

We have already referred specifically to self-surrender as the basic principle of femininity. Frigidity reveals that a woman is not prepared to give herself fully, but wants to 'wear the trousers' herself. She does not want to submit or be the 'underdog'; she wants to dominate. Such urges towards dominance and fantasies of power are expressions of the masculine principle, and therefore get in the way of the woman's full self-identification with her female role. By their very nature such displacements will disturb any polar process as sensitive as sexuality. This point is further confirmed by the fact that women who are frigid with their partners are perfectly capable of achieving orgasm by masturbating. In the case of masturbation the problem of dominating or giving oneself to another simply falls away – one is alone and needs to let nothing and nobody in apart from one's own fantasies. An 'I' that does not see itself as threatened by a 'you' finds it easier to withdraw willingly into the background. What also generally shows up in frigidity is women's fear of their own natural drives, especially in the presence of such strong value-judgements as are represented by clichés such as the 'respectable woman' or the 'whore'. The frigid woman wants to let nothing in or out, but merely to 'stay cool'.

The principle underlying masculinity is that of 'making', 'creating' and 'manifestation'. The masculine (yang) is active and, by the same token, aggressive. Potency is the expression and symbol of power, while impotence is lack of power. Behind impotence stands fear of one's own manhood and aggression. One is afraid of 'having to stand up for oneself'. Impotence also expresses a fear of femininity as such. The feminine is regarded as something that threatens to gobble one up. Here the feminine reveals itself in its aspect as the all-devouring Great Mother or witch. One wants at all costs to avoid entering the 'witch's cave'. At the same time we see here a minimal self-identification with the masculine and thus with attributes such as power and aggression. The impotent man tends to identify himself much more with the passive pole and thus with the submissive role. He is actually afraid of achievement. Here, then, the vicious circle begins once more as he attempts to achieve potency by sheer effort and will-power. The greater the pressure to perform, the less the prospect of an erection. Rather should impotence, then, serve as a cue to take stock of one's attitudes to such themes as power, achievement and aggression, and to the fears that are associated with them.

In considering sexual problems generally, meanwhile, we should never forget that in every human being there is both a feminine and a masculine psychological aspect, and that each of us, whether man or woman, needs to develop both of these inner aspects to the full. Nevertheless, this difficult path demands that we first achieve total identification with the particular aspect that is represented by our physical gender. Only when we are capable of living out that one pole to the full is the way free for us to awaken – and so to integrate consciously – the alternative aspect of our psyche via the encounter with the opposite sex.

Ten

The Heart and Circulation

Low and High Blood-Pressure (Hypotonia and Hypertonia)

Blood symbolises life. The blood is the physical vehicle of life and the expression of our individuality. The blood is not just 'a very special juice' – it is our very life-juice. Every drop of blood contains the whole person – hence the great significance of blood in magical practices. That is why pendulum-dowsers use drops of blood as 'witnesses': it is also why a single drop of blood can be used to make an overall diagnosis.

The blood-pressure is an expression of a person's general dynamism. It arises out of the mutual effects of the behaviour of the liquid blood on the one hand and the behaviour of the limiting walls of the blood-vessels on the other. When considering the blood-pressure we always need to bear in mind these two mutually contradictory components: the fluid and the flowing on the one hand and the limitation and the resistance of the walls of the blood-vessels on the other. To the extent that the blood corresponds to our own inner being, the walls of the blood-vessels correspond to the limits that the unfolding personality sets itself and the resistances that stand in the way of our development.

People with too low a blood-pressure (hypotonia) are failing totally to challenge those limits. They are making no attempt to stand on their own two feet, but ducking every resistance that stands in their way: they never take things to the limit. If they run into a conflict, they quickly withdraw: and by the same token the blood, too, withdraws, right up to the point where they actually lose consciousness. And so they (apparently) renounce all power, withdraw both their blood and their consciousness, and lay both themselves and their responsibilities down. By becoming unconscious they withdraw from the conscious world into the unconscious and so have nothing more to do with the problems that face them. They are just not there any more. It is an operatic situation with which we are only too familiar: a lady is caught by her husband in an embarrassing situation, and at once drops down in a faint, whereupon all those involved are anxious to recall her to consciousness with the help of water, fresh air and smelling-salts. What, after all, is the use of even the best of conflicts if the person who is mainly responsible withdraws to another level and thus resigns all responsibility at a stroke?

People with hypotonia are literally 'unable to stand': they cannot *stand* the pace, they will not *stand* up for anybody or anything, they lack steadfastness and *up-stand-ingness*. They will lie down in the face of every challenge, whereupon those around them will hoist their legs in the air so that more blood will flow back into their heads – their power-centres – and they can thus regain power over themselves and resume their responsibilities. Sexuality, too, is one of the areas that those with low blood-pressure tend to dodge, for sexuality is highly dependent on the blood-pressure.

In addition, we often find in those with hypotonia the symptomatology of anaemia, the commonest form of which involves a lack of iron in the blood. As a result, the transformation into physical energy of the cosmic energy (prana) that we take in as we breathe is disturbed. Anaemia reveals a refusal to take in the ration of life-energy to which we are entitled and to turn it into active force. Here again, illness is used as an alibi for our own passivity. We lack the necessary drive.

All the sensible therapeutic measures for raising the blood-pressure are coupled more or less without exception to various methods for injecting energy into the situation, and work only so long as the following prescriptions are persisted with: washings, brushings, treading water, movement, keep-fit exercises and the application of Kneipp (hydropathic) therapies. These raise the blood-pressure for the simple reason that the patient is actually *doing something* and thereby transforming energy into active force. They lose all their usefulness, however, the moment these exercises are abandoned. Lasting success is to be expected only from a change of inner attitude.

The opposite problem is represented by too high a blood-pressure (hypertonia). We know from experimental research that the pulse and blood-pressure are raised not just by increased physical activity, but simply by thinking about it. The blood-pressure likewise goes up if a conversation gets too close to a person's particular conflict area, but soon goes down again if the person concerned starts talking about the conflict of his or her own volition and so verbalises the problem involved. This experimentally based piece of knowledge offers us a good foundation for understanding what lies behind high blood-pressure. If constantly thinking about a given activity increases the circulation without the activity ever being translated into actual motor functions and so being discharged in physical form, what results is literally a kind of 'long-term pressure'. In this case those concerned produce within themselves a long-term excitation induced by their own imagination, and the circulatory system maintains this long-term excitation in the expectation that it will eventually be translated into action. If the action fails to materialise, the patient stays 'under pressure'. Of even greater importance to us here is the fact that the same relationship applies where conflict is concerned. Since we know that the theme of conflict can itself lead to a rise in pressure which can nevertheless be reversed merely by talking about it, we can see clearly that those with hypertonia are hanging around in the vicinity of various conflicts without applying any solution. They are 'standing next to' the conflict, but failing to address it. The raised blood-pressure has its physiological justification precisely in temporarily supplying more energy so that the tasks and conflicts facing us can be dealt with more efficiently and energetically. If this happens, the applied solution uses up the excess energy, and the pressure sinks back to its normal value. But those with hypertonia fail to resolve their conflicts, and the result is that the excess pressure is not used up. Rather do they take refuge in superficial 'busy-ness', attempting through great external activity to divert both themselves and others from the challenge actually to get to grips with the conflict.

We can readily see, then, that not only people whose blood-pressure is too low, but also those with high blood-pressure are avoiding impending conflicts, while at the same time using quite different tactics from each other. Those with hypotonia are taking refuge from conflict in a withdrawal into the unconscious: those with hypertonia, by contrast, are diverting both themselves and those around them away from the conflict through overactivity and exaggerated dynamism. In other words they are taking refuge in sheer action. Reflecting this polarity, we find low blood-pressure more frequently in women, but high blood-pressure more frequently in men. Furthermore, high blood-pressure is a sign of frustrated aggression. All the hostility gets stuck at the conceptual level, and so the available energy is not discharged in the form of action. Those concerned generally refer to this attitude as 'self-restraint'. The aggressive impulse raises the pressure, while the self-restraint leads to a contraction of the blood-vessels to keep the pressure under control. The pressure of the blood and the counter-pressure of the walls of the blood-vessels thus combine to produce high blood-pressure. We shall see in due course how this attitude of controlled aggression eventually leads directly to heart-attacks.

Also well-known is the form of high blood-pressure that is determined by age and goes with furring-up of the artery-walls. The arterial system's function is transmission and communication. To the extent that all flexibility and elasticity disappears with age, communication similarly becomes fossilised, and so the inner pressure inevitably rises.

The Heart

The beating of the heart is a largely autonomous activity which in the absence of certain kinds of training (such as biofeedback) is beyond the reach of voluntary intervention. This sinus rhythm represents a strict bodily norm. The rhythm of the heart resembles that of the breath, but with the latter much more amenable to deliberate intervention. The heartbeat is a strictly controlled harmonic rhythm. When the heart suddenly stumbles or races as a result of so-called rhythmic disturbances, it reveals a breach of the normal order – a departure from the normal symmetry.

On considering the many speech-idioms in which the heart figures, we can see that it always relates to emotional situations. An 'emotion' is something that we bring out of ourselves from within, a movement outwards from inside ourselves (Latin *emovere* = 'to move out of oneself'). We say such things as 'Her heart leaped for joy' – 'My heart was in my boots' – 'His heart was bursting with emotion' – 'My heart was in my mouth' – 'I've something on my heart' – 'She was close to his heart' – 'He takes it very much to heart.' If a person lacks this emotional aspect that is quite independent of reason, he or she strikes us as 'heartless'. When two lovers meet we speak of 'their hearts being as one'. In all these expressions the heart is used as a symbol for that centre within us that is conditioned neither by intellect nor by will.

Yet it is not just *a* centre, but *the* centre of the body: it lies virtually in the middle of it, only a little displaced to the left towards the 'feeling' side (corresponding to the brain's right hemisphere). Thus it lies exactly at the spot that we point to when we want to indicate *ourselves*. Feelings, and love in particular, are intimately bound up with the heart, as the many idioms already quoted make clear. If 'our heart goes out' to children, it means that we love them. If we 'hold somebody dear to our heart' we open ourselves to them and let them in. We are then 'big-hearted' people. We are prepared to open ourselves and our hearts to others: we are 'open-hearted'. In direct contrast are those who are reserved and 'heartless' – people who will not 'listen to their hearts', who know no 'heartfelt' feelings, but rather are 'cold-hearted'. They would never 'give their heart to another', for this would mean giving their very selves: on the contrary, they take every care not to 'put their heart into anything', and consequently do everything 'half-heartedly'. 'Soft-hearted' people, on the other hand, are prepared to risk loving others 'with all their heart', unreservedly and eternally. But then at least such feelings tend to point the way out of polarity, which demands that everything should have ends and limits.

We find both possibilities duly symbolised in the heart. The anatomical organ is divided into two by the heart's inner dividing-wall, just as the heartbeat itself is characterised by a double sound. For at birth, in the very moment when we draw our first breath and thus enter into polarity, the dividing-wall closes automatically by reflex action, and the *one* great chamber and the *one* circulation suddenly become *two* – an experience which often drives the newborn to *dis-traction*. Then again, the basic symbolism of the heart – just as any child would spontaneously draw it – can be further traced in its characteristic design, with its two rounded chambers joining together to form a single point. Out of two-ness grows oneness. And so it is that the heart is also a symbol for us of love and unity. That is what we mean when we say that a mother 'carries her child in her heart'. Taken anatomically, this expression would of course be senseless: here the heart is simply serving as a symbol for our love-centre, and so it matters not in the slightest that it lies anatomically in the upper half of the body, while the foetus does its growing lower down.

We could even say that we human beings have two centres: an upper one and a lower one – head and heart, understanding and feeling. We expect of a 'whole' person that the two functions should both be present and in harmonious balance. The purely intellectual person comes across as one-sided and cold, while people who live only from their feelings come across as rather muddled and confused. Only when both functions mutually complement and fructify each other does a person strike us as being 'rounded'.

The numerous expressions in which the heart is mentioned

make it clear to us that what disturbs the heart from its usual, regular beat is always some emotion – be it the shock that starts the heart racing or brings it to a standstill, or the joy or love that speed up the heartbeat to such an extent that we can hear and feel our heart beating in our very throat. The same thing happens where rhythmic disturbances of the heart are concerned – but in this case the corresponding emotion is nowhere to be seen. This indeed is where the problem lies: it is precisely on those people who are not prepared to be dragged by 'any old emotion' out of their familiar rut that such rhythmic disturbances tend to descend. In such cases the heart becomes disturbed because those concerned lack the confidence to let themselves be disturbed by their emotions. They cling on to their reason and their familiar way of life and are not ready to have their established routine disrupted by feelings and emotions. They do not want to have the harmonious regularity of their lives disturbed by emotional outbursts. Yet in such cases the emotion simply somatises itself, and the heart then starts disturbing them on its own account. The heartbeat goes wild and so forces those concerned literally to 'listen to their hearts'.

Under normal circumstances we are unaware of our heartbeat: we can hear and feel it only under the stress of emotion or illness. Our heartbeat comes to our conscious attention only when something is exciting us or when deep changes are afoot. Here, then, we have discovered the primary key to understanding all our heart-symptoms: heart-symptoms force us to 'listen to our hearts' once again. Heart patients are people who only want to listen to their heads, and in whose lives the heart figures far too little. This phenomenon is particularly obvious in cardiophobics. By 'cardiophobia' (or 'cadioneurosis') is meant a physically unfounded fear about the activity of one's own heart, which can lead to morbidly exaggerated attention being paid to the heart. Fears about the heartbeat can reach such a pitch in cardioneurotics that they are prepared to re-jig their whole lives purely on that account.

On considering this form of behaviour, we can see once again the degree of wisdom and irony with which illness operates. Cardiophobics are forced constantly to observe their hearts and to subordinate their entire lives to the needs of their hearts. In the process they live in constant fear of their hearts – or rather in the entirely valid fear that their hearts will one day stop and so leave them 'heartless'. The cardiophobia forces them to restore their hearts to the very centre of their conscious attention. And who could fail to laugh 'heartily' at that?

What in the cardioneurotic is happening at the psychological level is a process that in the case of *angina pectoris* has already descended deep into physicality. The blood-vessels leading to the heart have become hardened and constricted, so that it no longer receives sufficient nutrients. There is really not all that much interpretation to be done at this point, since everybody knows what to expect of people with 'hardened' and 'stony' hearts. The word *angina* literally means 'tightness', and *angina pectoris* thus means 'tight-chestedness'. Whereas the cardioneurotic is still experiencing this tightness directly in the form of fear, in the case of *angina pectoris* the tightness has gone on to manifest itself in concrete form. And at this point orthodox therapy comes up with a highly original piece of symbolism: in emergency, heart patients are given nitroglycerine capsules (such as Nitrolingual, for example) – in other words, explosives! In this way the tightness is 'blown apart', so as to create space for the heart once more in the patient's life. Heart patients in general are worried about their hearts – and rightly so!

Yet so many of us still fail to understand the challenge. Once the fear of personal feelings has reached such a pitch that we can no longer trust anything other than what is 'normal', we go and have a heart-pacemaker fitted. In this way the living rhythm is replaced by what is in effect a metronome (metre is to rhythm as *dead* is to *living*!) What previously was controlled by the feelings is now taken over by a machine. And while admittedly we lose the flexibility and adaptiveness of the natural heart-rhythm, at least the irregularities of a living heart no longer pose any threat to us. Those of us who are 'tight-hearted' have, in effect, become victims of our own egotistical urges and power-dreams.

Everybody knows that high blood-pressure is a predisposing factor for heart attacks. We have already seen that sufferers from hypertonia are people with a good deal of aggression who nevertheless keep it all in by exercising self-restraint. It is this blockage of aggressive energy that is released in a heart attack: it literally tears the heart apart. The heart attack is the sum of all the 'attacks' and 'beatings' that the patient has failed to mete out in the past. In a heart attack, consequently, we can experience at first hand the age-old teaching that to overvalue the powers of the ego and the dominance of the will is to cut ourselves off from the flow of the living. Only a hard heart can break!

HEART CONDITIONS

With heart disturbances and cardiac conditions, the following questions are well worth going into:

1. Are my head and heart, my intellect and feelings in harmonious balance?
2. Am I giving enough scope to my feelings and trusting myself to express them?
3. Am I living and loving 'heartily', or only 'half-heartedly'?
4. Is my life borne along by a living rhythm, or am I subjecting it to a regular, rigid measure?
5. Does my life still contain enough combustible materials and explosives?
6. Am I listening to my heart?

Weaknesses of the Connective Tissue – Varicose Veins – Thrombosis

The connective tissue (the mesenchyme) joins together all the specialised cells, gives them a firm basis and combines the individual organs and functional entities into a larger whole which we recognise as being a single unit. Weak connective tissue in a person reveals a lack of firmness, a tendency to compliance and a lack of inner resilience. Such people are as a rule easily wounded and somewhat resentful. In the body this syndrome shows up in the blue bruises that constantly appear at the slightest provocation.

The tendency to varicose veins is closely tied up with weakness of the connective tissue. In this case the blood collects in the superficial veins of the leg. As a result the circulation is overbalanced towards the lower human pole. This suggests that the person concerned has a pronounced earthy tendency, and indicates a certain sluggishness and cumbersomeness. Such people tend to lack resilience and elasticity. Virtually everything that we have said above in connection with anaemia and low blood-pressure also applies here.

Thrombosis is the blocking of a vein by a blood-clot. The real danger of thrombosis is that the clot may break loose and get into the lungs as an embolus. The problem underlying this symptom is easy to recognise. The blood, which by rights should be fluid and runny, solidifies, clots and congeals, so that the whole circulation stagnates. Fluidity presupposes a capacity for change. To the extent that we cease to change, symptoms arise in the body that have the effect of constricting and blocking in this context too. Outer mobility presupposes inner mobility. If our consciousness becomes sluggish and our opinions congeal into fixed views and judgements, that which in the bodily context should really be fluid also congeals. It is well-known that confinement to bed increases the risk of thrombosis. But confinement to bed also shows very clearly that the mobility-pole is no longer being lived out. 'Everything flows', said Heraclitus. In any polar form of existence, life shows up as movement and change. Every attempt to hang on exclusively to one of the two poles eventually leads to stagnation and death. That eternal state of being that is unchanging is to be found only beyond polarity. But to arrive at that point we have to trust ourselves to change, for it is only change that can ultimately bring us to that state which is unchangeable.

Eleven

The Motor System and Nerves

Attitude

When we speak of people's 'attitude' or 'stance' (to say nothing of their 'position', 'bearing' or 'posture') it is not immediately obvious from the expression itself whether we are referring to their physical attitude or to their inner attitude. However, this linguistic ambiguity does not of itself lead to any real misunderstanding, since our outer attitude in fact corresponds to our inner one. The outer is merely a mirror of the inner. Thus we speak, for example, of an 'upright' person, for the most part without being aware of the fact that the very idea of uprightness refers to a physical act which in the event was to prove of decisive importance in the history of humanity. No animal can be 'upright', for the simple reason that it has not yet achieved physical uprightness. Yet at some point in the dim and distant past humanity did manage to take the giant step of standing upright, and thus of turning its gaze upwards to the heavens and gaining the opportunity to become a god – while at the same time conjuring up the spectre of hubris, of already regarding itself as God with a capital 'G'. The simultaneous danger and opportunity inherent in standing upright is also evident on the purely physical level. The soft parts of the body, well-protected in a four-legged animal by its physical stance, are left unprotected when the human being stands upright. This defencelessness and increased vulnerability nevertheless brings with it as its polar counterpart a greater openness and sensitivity. It is specifically the spinal column which permits our upright stance. It makes us both straight and flexible, gives us both firmness and suppleness. It takes the form of a double-S, and works on the shock-absorber principle. It is the polarity between solid vertebrae on the one hand and soft intervertebral discs on the other that gives us our suppleness and flexibility.

We have already pointed out the direct correspondence between inner and outer attitude. This analogy is expressed in many a turn of speech. Thus, there are 'straight' and 'upright' folk, as well as those who are 'bent': we all know 'starchy' or 'stiff-necked' people, as well as others who are prepared to 'grovel' or 'cringe'. Many of us lack not only 'upstandingness', but any sort of 'firm footing' at all. Yet at the same time we can seek to influence our 'standing' by making a pretence at a particular inner attitude. Thus it is that parents yell at their children, 'Stand up straight!', or 'Can't you ever sit straight, for heaven's sake?' And so the dishonesty game gets under way.

Later on it is the military who demand of their troops that they 'take up position'. At this point, though, the situation starts to get truly grotesque. The individual soldier is expected to take up a particular stance, even though inwardly he is not allowed to have one. Ever since the year dot the military have drilled their troops at great expense to take up given stances, even though from the tactical point of view these are just plain idiotic. Neither goose-stepping nor standing to attention are of the slightest use in the hurly burly of battle. The only reason for training soldiers to take up particular stances and positions is to break the natural correspondence between inward and outward attitude. Whereupon the fact that the soldiery inwardly lack the approved outer attitude comes straight out into the open the moment they are off duty, after a victory or on other, similar occasions. Guerrilla fighters have no need to take up outward stances or attitudes because they are inwardly identified with what they are doing. Our effectiveness increases perceptibly in line with our inner attitude, and decreases with artificially imposed external ones. We could contrast, for example, the rigid attitude of a soldier, standing to attention with straight arms and legs, with that of a cowboy, who would never dream of restricting his mobility by keeping his arms and legs straight. This open attitude which allows one to find one's own centre of gravity is also to be found in Tai Chi.

We immediately recognise as unnatural any attitude that does not correspond to a person's inner nature, yet we can also recognise a natural attitude in anybody. If illness forces somebody into a particular position that he or she would never willingly take up, this position reveals to us an inner attitude that is not being lived out – one that the person concerned is actually fighting against.

In considering individual people, then, we need to decide whether they are truly identified with their surface attitude, or whether they are being made to take up that attitude against their will. In the first case their attitude simply reflects the way in which they consciously identify themselves. In the latter case what shows up in their pathologically altered attitude is some shadow-area that they in fact want nothing to do with. Thus, people who stride through life extremely straight and upright, and with head held high, contrive to convey a certain haughtiness, pride, loftiness and uprightness. But such people will also find it quite easy to identify with all these qualities. They will simply not deny them.

It is quite a different matter, however, where ankylosing spondylitis (*morbus Bechterew*) is concerned, with its characteristic bamboo-like deformation of the spinal column. This represents a somatisation of unconscious egotism and of an inflexibility of which the patient is totally unaware. In this disease the spinal column eventually ossifies into a single piece, the back becomes stiff and the head is pushed forward as a result of the spine's S-shape being straightened out or even reversed. Patients almost literally have their noses rubbed in the fact that they are really stiff, unyielding and inflexible. The problem area that manifests itself in a hunched back is very similar: the hump is a manifestation of a submissiveness that the patient is failing to live out in practice.

The Vertebral Discs and Sciatica

Under pressure, the cartilaginous discs between the vertebrae – and especially those in the area of the lumbar vertebrae – are squeezed out sideways and press against the nerves, so causing various types of pain such as sciatica, lumbago and so on. The problem underlying this symptomatology is that of *overburdening oneself*. Those who heap too much on their own shoulders and are not consciously aware of this excess duly experience the resulting pressure in the body in the form of back-pain. The pain forces them to take things easy, for every movement, every activity hurts. A good many people try to suppress this perfectly sensible piece of self-regulation with the aid of pain-killers, so that they can carry on regardless with their regular activities. But it would actually be far more sensible for them to take the opportunity quietly to think over why they have taken on so much and thus laid such pressure on themselves. In fact, taking on too much is always a way of trying to look big and competent, so as to compensate by our actions for feeling small inside.

Behind great achievements there always stand feelings of insecurity and inferiority. People who have truly discovered themselves no longer need to achieve anything: they just *are*. Nevertheless, behind all the great (and not so great) achievements of world history there always stand people who have been spurred on to outward greatness by feelings of inner inferiority. They are determined to prove something to the world by what they do, notwithstanding the fact that there is nobody there to demand or expect any such proof – apart from themselves, that is. They are constantly trying to prove something *to themselves*. The question, though, is 'What?' Such over-achievers would do well to take the earliest opportunity to ask themselves just why they are doing it all, so that the eventual let-down does not hit them too hard. Those who are honest with themselves will eventually discover that the answer is, 'To be recognised, to be loved.' Yet, true though it is that the search for love is the only known motivation for achievement, the quest always ends in disillusion, for the goal is actually unattainable via this route. Love, after all, is motiveless, and is not something that can be earned. 'I will love you if you give me a thousand pounds,' or 'I love you because you are the best footballer' are absurd statements. The secret of love resides precisely in its unconditionality. Thus, the prototype of love is to be found in a mother's love. From the objective point of view, all that the baby brings its mother is trouble and inconvenience. Yet that is not how the mother sees it, for she loves her baby. Why? There is no answer. If there were, it would not be love. Consciously or unconsciously, we all long for a love that is pure, unconditional, self-validating and totally independent of all externals and personal achievements.

What feelings of inferiority amount to, then, is a conviction that we are unlovable as we are. And so we start trying to make ourselves lovable by becoming more and more clever, competent, rich, famous and so on. With all this outer tinsel we aim to make ourselves lovable – yet if we now discover that people *do* love us, we start to wonder whether we are 'only' being loved for our achievements, our fame, our money or whatever. We ourselves have contrived to block the way to true love. The fact that our achievements are recognised does not even satisfy the desire that drove us to them in the first place. That is why it is useful to come to terms consciously with our own feelings of inferiority and smallness in good time. Those of us who refuse to recognise what is involved, and who insist on heaping yet further tasks on themselves, actually start at this point to get physically smaller. As a result of the compression of the spinal discs they start to shrink, and the pain makes them take up crooked, bent attitudes. The body always tells the truth.

The discs' job is to preserve our suppleness and elasticity. If vertebrae that are wedged together cause a disc to jam and its movement to become inhibited, our attitude, too, becomes stiff and immobile and we often take up peculiar positions. The self-same pattern crops up in the psychological realm, too. If we are psychologically inhibited, we lack all openness and flexibility – we are stiff, and insist on maintaining a particular inner attitude. In chiropractic, jammed discs are freed by releasing the vertebrae from their wedged positions with the aid of a sudden push or pull, so making it possible for them to come back into natural contact with each other again (*solve et coagula*).

In the same way inhibited souls, too, are best 'set right' or 'straightened out' along much the same lines as joints and vertebrae. They need to be jolted out of their existing position with the aid of a sudden, hard push if they are to have any chance of reorientating and rediscovering themselves. Those who are inhibited are just as afraid of being jolted in this way as are patients of being manipulated by the chiropractor. In both cases, though, it is a sharp crack that signals the prospect of real success.

The Joints

It is the joints that make us mobile. Many of the symptoms that affect the joints lead via inflammation to pain, with this leading in turn to restrictions on movement and even a total stiffening up. When a joint does stiffen up, this is a sign that the patient has 'taken up a rigid stance' in respect of something or other. A stiffened joint loses its function: by the same token, then, if we take up a rigid stance on any question or system, this likewise loses its functional value for us. A stiff neck does indeed show us that its owner is figuratively stiff-necked. It is generally quite sufficient to listen to the words we use to find out what any given symptom is telling us. In addition to inflammation and stiffening, joints are also subject to sprains, strains, bruising and torn ligaments. Here again, the associated figures of speech are highly revealing. In the present case we need only mull over in our minds such phrases as the following: to 'overstretch ourselves' – to 'go too far' – to 'put a strain on somebody' – to 'put somebody under pressure' – to 'become over-tense or over-strained' – even to 'get all screwed up'. It is not only joints that we can 'set right' or 'straighten out', but also situations, relationships and states of affairs.

Resetting a joint often involves bending it into an extreme

position, or extending even further its current extreme position, so that it can return from that extreme to its new mid-point. This technique has its direct counterpart in psychotherapy, too. If somebody is stuck in an extreme sitting position, it is possible to force them even further into that position until they finally reach a turning-point from which they are able to rediscover the 'happy medium'. The quickest way out of any given position is to get right to the heart of the pole in question. But cowardice generally prevents us adopting as whole-hearted an approach as this, and so we get stuck half-way with the particular pole in question. Because most people only ever do things by halves, they get bogged down in their own views and familiar ways of behaving, and too little real change results. Yet every pole has a limiting value at which it turns into its opposite. Thus, extreme tension is a very good way of achieving relaxation (Jakobsen training). That is why physics was the first of the sciences to discover metaphysics. It is also why peace movements tend to become militant. The happy medium is something that has to be worked for: any attempt to grasp it directly merely gets bogged down in mediocrity.

Nevertheless mobility, too, can be overdone to such an extent that it turns into immobility. The mechanical changes that appear in our joints often reveal these limits to us, and show us that we have exploited one particular pole or direction so exhaustively that its own continued existence is being thrown into question. In other words we have gone too far and overdone things, and so the time has now come to turn our attention to the opposite pole.

Modern medicine enables us to replace various joints with artificial prostheses. This happens particularly frequently in the case of the hip-joint (endoprosthesis). As we have already emphasised in connection with dentition, a prosthesis is always a deception, in that a pretence is being made that something is there when it is not. If a person is inwardly stiff and rigid, yet behaves in such a way as to make an outward show of mobility, the hip-symptom corrects the situation by injecting greater honesty into it. The effect of an artificial hip-joint, however, is to cancel out this correction by once again giving the impression of physical mobility.

In order to gain an impression of just how dishonest medicine enables us to be, let us mentally imagine the following situation: just assume that it were possible suddenly to magic away all the artificial prostheses that people have – their glasses and contact-lenses, their hearing-aids, artificial joints, man-made teeth, facelifts, metal bone-pins, pacemakers, and all the other various bits of metal and plastic that people have had implanted. Imagine how horrendous the resulting sight would be!

Now let us cast a further magic spell and take back all the medical achievements that have saved people from dying in the past. Immediately we should be surrounded by corpses, cripples, the lame, the half-blind and the half-deaf. It is a horrifying picture – yet at least it would be honest! It would be the visible expression of the true state of the human soul. A lot of medical skill has gone into sparing us this grisly prospect by zealously restoring the human body and building it up with so many artificial bits and pieces that in the end it almost looks alive and real. But what has become of people's souls in all this? Here nothing has changed. They are just as dead, blind, deaf, stiff, cramped or crippled as ever they were. It is just that we cannot see it. That is why we are so afraid of being honest. It is the story of *The Picture of Dorian Gray* all over again. We can use all kinds of trickery to preserve our youth and beauty for a while – but great is the horror as soon as we are faced with what we really look like inside. Constant work on our souls has to be far more important than just looking after our bodies, for the body is impermanent, whereas our consciousness is not.

Rheumatoid Conditions

Rheumatism is an ill-defined umbrella-term for a group of symptoms involving painful changes in the tissues which show up primarily in the joints and musculature. Rheumatism is always linked to inflammation, which can be either acute or chronic. It leads to swelling of the tissues or muscles and distortion and/or hardening of the joints. Patients' mobility can be so restricted by the pain that they can be turned into invalids. The pain in the joints and muscles gets worse after periods of rest and improves with exercise. Inactivity leads in time to a wasting of the muscles. It also leads eventually to a spindle-shaped distension of the joints affected.

The illness generally starts with morning stiffness and painful joints: the latter swell up and often go red. The joints are normally affected symmetrically, while the pain tends to move inwards from the small, peripheral joints towards the large, main joints. The illness tends to be chronic, while the stiffness tends to increase by degrees.

The course of the illness leads via increasing stiffness to an ever more severe degree of incapacity. Nevertheless polyarthritics complain very little, showing great patience and displaying astonishing indifference to their sufferings.

The symptomatology of polyarthritis confronts us particularly vividly with the central theme of all illness of the motor system – namely the polarity between motion and rest, between mobility and rigidity. The personal history of nearly all rheumatic patients reveals excessive activity and mobility. Typically, they have engaged in competitive and combative sports, have worked hard at home and in the garden, have been tirelessly on the go all the time, and have made a point of sacrificing themselves for others. It is thus on active, mobile, agile, restless people that polyarthritis inflicts its long-term stiffness and rigidity, right up to the point where disablement finally forces them to keep still. What seems to be happening here, in other words, is that excessive movement and activity is being corrected for by means of rigidity.

This may at first sight seem surprising, in view of our constant insistence hitherto on the need for change and movement. The link only becomes clear when we recall once again that the function of bodily illness is to force us to be honest. In the case of polyarthritis, this would imply that the people concerned are actually quite rigid. The overactivity and excessive mobility which always seems to precede the illness unfortunately only applies in the physical context, and is merely a compensation for a consciousness that is actually in the grip of immobility. In German, for example, the word *starr* (rigid) is closely related to the words *stur* (stubborn), *steif* (stiff), *störrisch* (obstinate) and even *stieren* (to stare) and *sterben* (to die).

These terms all fit very closely the typology of the polyarthritic patient, whose characteristic personality-type is extremely well known, thanks to the fact that psychosomatic medicine has been researching this particular group of patients for a good half-century now. Thus, researchers are universally agreed that (to quote Bräutigam once again), 'the character of the polyarthritic patient shows a compulsive tendency towards over-conscientiousness and perfectionism, as well as a masochistic/depressive tendency with a strong need for self-sacrifice and exaggerated helpfulness, combined with excessively moral behaviour and a proneness to depressive moods.' These character traits show how rigid and stubborn, how inflexible and immobile of soul such people really are. All the sporting activity and physical restlessness merely serve to over-compensate for this inner immobility and divert attention from their compulsive rigidity by way of a defence-mechanism.

The remarkably frequent participation of such patients in various types of combative sport now brings us to their next focal problem area – namely aggression. Rheumatics tend to inhibit their aggression on the motor level – in other words, they block their energy at the muscular stage. Experimental tapping and measurement of the electrical activity in the muscles of rheumatics has shown clearly that any kind of stimulus leads in their case to increased muscle-tension, especially in respect of the joint muscles. Such measurements merely serve to raise the obvious suspicion that rheumatics have a compulsion to restrain the various aggressive impulses that seek to translate themselves into physical action. The energy which remains undischarged in this way stays bottled up and unused in the joint muscles, where it is transformed into inflammation and pain. Every pain that we undergo in the course of illness is a pain that was originally intended for somebody else. Pain is always the result of some piece of aggression. If I give free rein to my aggression by hitting somebody else, it is my victim who feels the pain. If, on the other hand, I restrain my aggressive impulse, it turns on me instead, and I am the one who feels the pain (auto-aggression). Anybody who suffers from aches and pains should always reflect on just who those pains were really intended for.

In the rheumatoid family there is one symptom in particular that involves the hand clenching itself into a fist (chronic epicondylopathy) as a result of inflammation of the ligaments of the muscles of the forearm at the elbow. The resulting image of the 'clenched fist' shows vividly patients' bottled-up aggression and their repressed desire to 'bang their fists on the table'. A similar tendency to turn the hand into a fist can be seen in Dupuytren's contracture, in which the hand can no longer be opened at all. The open hand, by contrast, is a symbol of peaceableness. Greeting people by saluting them with the hand goes back to the custom of showing the people we meet our open, empty hand so that they can see that we are holding no weapon in it and that we are approaching them with peaceful intentions. The same symbolism applies when we 'offer somebody a hand'. Just as the open hand is an expression of peaceful and conciliatory intentions, so the clenched fist remains a sign of hostility and aggression.

Rheumatics cannot admit to their own aggressive impulses. Otherwise, clearly, they would not repress and block them. Since, however, those impulses are still there, they produce strong unconscious guilt-feelings, which in turn lead them to display great helpfulness and self-sacrifice on behalf of others.

The result is that strange combination of altruistic service and simultaneous domination of others which Alexander described in the apt phrase 'benevolent dictatorship'. Often it is precisely when some change in life-circumstances deprives those concerned of the chance to use service to compensate for their guilt-feelings that the illness puts in its appearance. Rheumatism's repertory of most frequent side-effects likewise reveals to us how central to it repressed aggression is: foremost among these symptoms, after all, are gastric and intestinal ailments, heart-symptoms, frigidity and problems of sexual potency, to say nothing of anxiety and depression. Even the fact that around twice as many women as men are affected by polyarthritis is presumably explicable in terms of the fact that women tend to feel more inhibited about consciously acting out their hostile impulses.

Naturopathy traces rheumatism back to an accumulation of toxins in the connective tissue. From our own viewpoint as expressed in this book, accumulated toxins symbolise untackled problems or undigested themes which the patient has bottled up in the unconscious rather than resolving them. This is where the whole point of fasting comes in.* With the total removal of external food-sources, the organism switches over to its own food-supply, and so is forced among other things to burn up and process the contents of the body's own 'dustbin'. This process corresponds on the psychological level to working on the subject areas which have hitherto been pushed under and repressed, and to bringing them into the full light of consciousness. But rheumatics just do not want to address their problems. They are too rigid and immobile – in fact they have long since 'taken up a rigid stance' towards them. They are far too scared to subject their altruism, their servility and unselfishness, their moral standards and general complaisance to honest investigation. And so their egotism, their immobility, their inability to adapt, their urge to dominate and their aggression all remain hidden in the shadows, from where they subsequently go on to somatise themselves in the body as a stiffness and immobility that is perfectly obvious to everybody, so finally putting paid to all the false servility.

Motor Disturbances: Wryneck and Writer's Cramp

The common trademark of these disturbances is that patients partially lose control of motor functions that are normally

Compare Dahlke, R.: Bewußt Fasten (Urania, Waakirchen, 1980).

subject to their conscious will. Certain of these functions are particularly prone to escape voluntary control and generally go haywire when patients are aware of being observed or find themselves in situations where they are anxious to make an impression on others. Thus, in wryneck (*torticollis spasticus*) the head turns either slowly or violently to one side, to the point where it is almost totally averted. In most cases it can then be brought back to its normal position within a few seconds. It is notable that certain mechanical aids, such as placing the finger on the chin or using a neck-support, can make it easier for patients to hold their head straight. What has a particular influence on the configuration of the neck, however, is patients' own subjective assessment of their spatial situation. If they stand with their back to the wall so that they can lean their head against it, they generally have no difficulty in holding the head straight.

This peculiarity, as well as the symptom's dependence on particular situations (and specifically the presence of other people), shows us straight away what the main problem underlying all these disturbances is: it revolves around the polarity between security and insecurity. The motor disturbances affecting otherwise voluntary functions – including all the various tics – reveal how anxious those involved are to make a show of self-confidence for the benefit of others, while at the same time betraying the fact that they not only have no such confidence, but that they do not even have power or control over themselves. It has always been regarded as a sign of courage and bravery to look other people full in the face with unflinching eyes. But in precisely those situations where it actually comes to applying this approach, wryneck sufferers' heads insist on turning aside under their own steam. As a result such people become more and more afraid to meet important people or to be seen socially – a fear that at least is honest. Because of the symptom they now go on to avoid certain situations in just the same way as they have always avoided other unpleasant situations. They avert their gaze from their various conflicts and let one side of life languish unseen on the sidelines.

Keeping the head and body erect forces us to look all our challenges straight in the eye and see them directly and immediately for what they are. If we turn our heads away, though, we are avoiding this confrontation. We become 'lop-sided' and turn away from whatever it is that we do not want to confront. We start to see things 'askew' and 'awry'. No doubt it is to this 'skew' and 'wry' way of looking at things that the well-known expression 'to turn a person's head' refers. Such a psychological affliction also has the aim of depriving victims of all control over where they actually look, and so of obliging them willy nilly to follow others with their eyes and thoughts.

We find a very similar background where writer's cramp and the finger-cramps of pianists and violinists are concerned. In such patients' personalities we always find extreme pride and an inordinate degree of pretension. Those affected are deliberately aiming to advance themselves socially, while at the same time making a superficial show of great modesty. They are anxious to impress others purely by their performance (by their beautiful writing or their music). The symptomatology of tonic cramping of the hand thus leads to honesty: it shows the almost 'convulsive' nature of patients' efforts and performances, and makes it abundantly clear that in reality they 'have nothing to say' (or to write).

Nail-Biting

While admittedly nail-biting is not a motor disturbance, we intend to deal with it here along with this particular group of conditions because of its superficial similarity to them. For nail-biting, too, is experienced as a kind of compulsion that overcomes the purely voluntary control of the hands. Not only does nail-biting crop up as a passing symptom among children and young people, but adults themselves often suffer for decades from this extremely hard-to-treat symptom. Yet the psychological background to nail-biting is perfectly clear, and recognising the links involved should thus be helpful to many a parent when this symptom appears in their children. For prohibitions, threats and punishments are, of all reactions, the least appropriate.

What in human beings we refer to as 'fingernails' are 'claws' where animals are concerned. The claws serve primarily for defence and attack: in other words, they are instruments of aggression. We speak of 'showing one's claws' in much the same sense as 'baring one's teeth'. An animal's claws show its willingness to fight. Indeed, the majority of the more advanced beasts of prey use their claws and teeth as weapons. Nail-biting, then, is the castration of one's own aggressive impulses! Nail-biters are afraid of their own aggression, and therefore symbolically blunt their own weapons. The biting itself helps to use up some of that aggression, yet it is directed exclusively against themselves: what they are actually biting off is their own aggression.

215

The main reason for women's suffering from symptomatic nail-biting is their envy of other women's long, red, varnished fingernails. Long nails, varnished in the martial colour of red are, after all, a particularly splendid, gleaming symbol of aggression: women who sport them are putting their aggressive disposition on open display for everybody to see. It is obvious, then, that such women will tend to be envied by others who do not trust themselves to admit to their own aggression and the weapons that go with it. Indeed, the very fact of wishing that they themselves had such long, red fingernails is merely the outward expression of their underlying wish that they, too, could be so openly aggressive.

Childhood nail-biting is a sign that the child concerned is at a stage where it lacks the confidence to give vent to its aggression. In this case parents should devote some thought to just how far they are repressing or attaching a negative value to aggressive behaviour via their own example or their methods of upbringing. In this event they should endeavour to give the child sufficient space to work up the courage to translate its aggressive impulses or guilt-feelings into action. Generally, of course, doing anything of the kind will generate a good deal of anxiety in the parents, for if they themselves had no problems with their own aggression they would have no nail-biting offspring either. Consequently it would be a healthy development for the whole family if they started to question their own dishonest and hypocritical ways of behaving and so learnt to see what is really lurking behind the whole façade. Once the child has learnt to stand up for itself instead of kowtowing to its parents' fears, the nail-biting too will itself be as good as overcome. All the while parents are not prepared to change themselves, they should at least not complain about their children's symptomatic disturbances. It is not that parents are to blame for their children's disturbances: it is merely that children's disturbances reflect the problems of their parents!

Stuttering

Speech is something that flows: we speak of the 'flow of conversation' and of a 'flowing style'. In stutterers, however, the flow of speech is interrupted. They cut it apart, chop it up, dismember it. If anything is to flow, it needs elbow-room: if, after all, we were to force water through a nozzle, congestion and pressure would build up, and the water would at best squirt out of the nozzle rather than simply flowing. Stutterers, similarly, inhibit the flow of speech by constricting their throats. We have already pointed out that constriction and fear always go together. In stutterers that fear is localised in the throat – which is both the link (already quite narrow in itself) and the communicating door between body and head, between below and above.

At this point we should do well to recall everything we said about the symbolism of 'Below' and 'Above' in the earlier chapter on migraine. Stutterers are people who are trying to make the throat's connecting door as narrow as possible so that they can exercise extra-tight control over what comes up from below – or, by analogy, over what is trying to emerge out of the unconscious into the conscious mind. It is the same defensive strategy that we can see in ancient fortifications, with their quite small and easily defendable passageways. What makes such entrances (both external and internal) so easy to control is the fact that they tend to get jammed solid, so hindering the flow of bodies through them. Stutterers, similarly, exercise their control in the throat because they are afraid of what is coming up from below and trying to become conscious: in other words, they 'take it by the throat' and throttle it.

We are all familiar with the phrase 'below the belt'. What this actually refers to, of course, is the 'indecent and smutty' subject of sexuality. The 'belt' represents the borderline between the 'dangerous' lower level and the 'clean', 'approved' upper realm. What stutterers have done is to shift this borderline up to the neck-level, thanks to their sense that everything to do with the body is dangerous and that only the head is pure and clean. Just like migraine patients, stutterers displace their sexuality up into their heads, with the result that they get just as screwed up at the higher level as at the lower. They refuse to let go or open themselves up to the body's drives and urges, whose pressure becomes all the greater and all the more frightening to them the longer they suppress them. What is more, they eventually go on to invoke their stuttering-symptom as the *cause* of all their difficulties of relationship and/or partnership – and so the vicious circle duly closes once again.

By a similar trick of distortion, the inhibitions which are always to be found in stuttering children are likewise normally interpreted as consequences of the stuttering. Yet the stuttering is in fact merely an expression of the inhibition – that is, the child is inhibited, and it is this that duly shows up in the stuttering. Children who stutter are afraid to give vent to some pressing matter, fearful of giving it free rein. They restrict the flow the better to control it. It is of no great consequence whether we identify that pressing matter as sexuality and aggression or prefer to substitute other labels in the light of individual circumstances. Stutterers are simply avoiding saying right out what comes to them. Speech is a means of expression. But if we put pressures in the way of what is trying to get out, what we are really doing is showing our *fear* of what is trying to get out. In consequence, we cease to be open. Once stutterers do manage to open themselves up, a violent torrent of sex, aggression and sheer words comes pouring out. Once everything unsaid has been said, after all, there is no more reason to stutter.

Twelve

Accidents

Many people react with great astonishment to the very idea of interpreting accidents in the same way as other illnesses. It is somehow assumed that accidents are a quite different kettle of fish: after all, it is argued, accidents ultimately come from 'out there', so we ourselves can hardly be to blame for them. Arguments of this sort show again and again how confused and inaccurate our thinking generally is – or rather how prone we are to suit our theoretical thinking to what we ourselves unconsciously want. We find it highly distasteful to take full responsibility for our existence as a whole and to take on board all the experiences that it brings to us. We are constantly on the lookout for chances to project our own blame 'out there'. We never fail to get angry when such projections are unmasked for what they are. Most of our scientific efforts are devoted to bolstering and justifying our own projections. From the human point of view, of course, this is all perfectly understandable. Yet since this book has been written for people who are looking for the truth, and who know that this goal can be attained only through honest self-knowledge, we cannot allow mere cowardice to stop us considering the topic of accidents.

We need to stay fully alive to the fact that there are always aspects of our experience that seem to come from 'out there', and that it is always possible to interpret these as 'causes'. This causal mode of interpretation, however, is only *one* possible way of considering the relationships between things: in this book we have decided to replace, or rather complement, this habitual approach with another that is just as possible. When we look in a mirror, the mirror-image, equally, seems to look at us from 'out there', and yet it is not the *reason* for the way we look. When we have a cold, it is the germs that come to us from 'out there', and so we see them in turn as the cause. If we are involved in a car-accident it is the drunken driver who comes out at us from the side-road, and so we naturally see him or her as the cause of the accident. There is always an explanation on the functional level. Yet this still does not stop us interpreting what happens in the light of its inner content.

The law of resonance sees to it that we never come into contact with anything that does not affect us directly. Functional relationships are simply the physical medium that is essential if any manifestation is to occur on the material level. In order to paint a picture we need canvas and paints – yet these are not the cause of the picture, but merely the physical media that the artist uses to realise his or her inner picture in formal terms. It would be stupid to dismiss an interpretation of what the picture is about by arguing that the real causes of the picture were the paints, canvas and brushes.

We shall be looking into the accidents that befall us, then, in just the same way as we have been looking into our 'illnesses', and in the process we shall not shrink from considering any matter merely so as to be able to treat it as a 'cause'. Quite the contrary – for the responsibility for everything that happens to us in life is always ours alone. To this there are no exceptions – and so we might just as well stop looking for any. To the extent that we suffer at all, it is always ourselves that we suffer from (which is not, of course, to deny the severity of the suffering). Each of us is perpetrator and victim rolled into one. All the while we fail to discover both of them within ourselves, there is no chance of our becoming whole. It is quite easy to tell from the intensity with which people blame the supposed perpetrators 'out there' how much they are still at odds with their own inner perpetrator. What is lacking here is *in-sight* – that sight which allows us to see that both perpetrator and victim are really within ourselves.

The knowledge that accidents are unconsciously motivated is far from new. Freud himself long ago suggested in his *Psychopathology of Everyday Life* that accidents, like slips of the tongue, forgetting, mislaying things and other 'Freudian slips', are actually the products of unconscious intentions. Since that time psychosomatic research has been able to demonstrate on purely statistical grounds the existence of a so-called 'accident-prone' personality-type. By this is meant a specific personality-structure that tends to work out its conflicts in the form of accidents. As early as 1926, the German psychologist K. Marbe published under the title *Praktische Psychologie der Unfälle und Betriebsschäden* his observation that a person who has suffered an accident is more likely to undergo further accidents than people who have never been accident-victims at all.

In the seminal work by Alexander on psychosomatic

medicine that came out in 1950 we find the following remarks on this topic: 'In the course of research into car-accidents in Connecticut it was shown that over a period of six years 36.4 per cent of all accidents occurred to a small group of 3.9 per cent of all those drivers involved in accidents. A large business concern employing numerous truck-drivers eventually became so concerned about the high cost of its vehicle-accidents that it had the causes of those accidents researched in an effort to reduce their frequency. Among other approaches they also did some research into the accident-history of individual drivers, and those who had had the most accidents were shifted to other jobs as a result. This simple measure succeeded in reducing the frequency of accidents to a fifth of its original value. But the really interesting outcome of this investigation is that those drivers with a high accident-quota remained just as liable to have accidents in their new jobs. This shows incontrovertibly that accident-prone people do really exist, and that individuals who tend to have accidents retain this characteristic in every type of employment, as well as in their daily life' (Alexander, F.: *Psychosomatic Medicine*).

Alexander further deduces that 'in most accidents an intentional element is involved, even though that intention is hardly ever conscious. In other words, most accidents are unconsciously motivated.' This foray into the more venerable archives of psychological literature should also demonstrate among other things that there is nothing new about our way of looking at accidents, however long it may take for such distasteful findings to penetrate the general consciousness (if, indeed, they ever do).

As we go on to consider the topic further, however, what will interest us is less describing the characteristic accident-personality as establishing the meaning of an accident when it happens to us in the actual course of our lives. Even if we ourselves do not display the typical accident-personality, the occurrence of an accident still has a meaning for us – and what we are anxious to do here is to learn how to discover that meaning. If accidents keep happening one after the other in a person's life, moreover, this is merely a sign that that person has failed to solve his or her problems on the conscious level, with the result that the forcible lessons go on escalating. The fact that particular people manifest their corrective experiences primarily in the form of accidents is a function of other people's *locus minoris resistentiae*. An accident throws its victim's way of doing things – indeed their whole chosen life-path to date – directly and abruptly into question. It is a break in their lives, and demands to be investigated as such. In the process they need to look at the whole history of the accident like a piece of theatre, endeavouring to understand the detailed structure of the circumstances that led to it, and to apply what they discover to their current situation. An accident is a caricature of one's problems – and just as penetrating and painful as any other caricature.

Traffic Accidents

So abstract is the general term 'traffic accident' that it is not possible to offer any overall interpretation of it. We need to know in detail what happens in a particular accident before we can say what underlying meaning is involved. Difficult or even impossible though it may be to arrive at a generalised interpretation, however, it is every bit as easy to interpret specific cases. It is sufficient to listen in carefully to how people describe what happened. The ambiguity of our language gives the whole game away. Unfortunately, though, one notices again and again that many people simply have no ear for such linguistic connections. In our practice, consequently, we often ask patients to keep repeating one particular sentence from their description until something rings a bell for them. On such occasions one never ceases to be amazed at people's unconscious gift for handling language, as well as at how efficient our critical filters are when it comes to masking our own particular problems.

Thus, in life as in the road-traffic context, we can, for example, 'lose our way' – 'get into a spin' – 'lose our grip' – 'lose control' – 'run off the road' – or, for that matter, 'run into somebody'. What more is there to interpret in such cases? It is sufficient to keep our ears open. Here, for example, we may have a man who is in such a hurry that he 'can't stop' and consequently not only 'gets too close' to the man (or is it a woman?) in front, but actually 'runs into him or her' so that they 'come into close (even intimate) contact' (or 'give each other a bang', as some people would prefer to put it). This powerful 'shock' is not unnaturally regarded as 'shocking'. Many drivers 'fly at each other' not merely with their cars, but in verbal terms too.

Quite often the question 'Who was to blame for the accident?' brings the standard answer 'I couldn't stop in time' – thus showing that those concerned are in such a tearing hurry over some personal life-development (a professional one, for example) that the development in question is actually starting to pose a threat to itself. Those concerned should take it as a summons to have a good look at all the rush in their lives and to slow down the pace in good time. 'I just didn't see him' is a clear indication that those concerned are overlooking something of real importance in their lives. If an attempt to overtake leads to an accident, it is time to re-examine all the 'overtaking manoeuvres' in one's own life at the earliest opportunity. People who fall asleep at the wheel need to wake up to what is happening in their lives, before they undergo some much ruder awakening. If we break down at night, we should look carefully at what things within the night-side of our soul could be bringing us to a halt. One person 'cuts in on' somebody else, a second 'infringes' road signs and markings, a third has to 'get himself out of the mire again'. Suddenly we cannot see clearly, we ignore stop-signs, we take the wrong direction, we bump into obstacles. Traffic-accidents nearly always lead to highly intensive contact with others – at least to people coming a good deal too close to one another – but always that approach is too aggressive.

At this point, then, let us consider and interpret together one specific road-accident by way of an example of how better to approach such an investigation. This particular case is not an invented one, though at the same time it corresponds to a very frequent type of traffic-accident. At a crossroads with priority to the right, two cars crash into each other with such violence that one of them is thrown onto the pavement, where it finishes up with all four wheels in the air. Several people are trapped inside, shouting for help. Loud radio-music blares from the car. Passers-by eventually manage to free the trapped victims from their metal prison. They are quite badly injured and finish up in hospital.

This train of events suggests the following interpretation: all the participants were in a situation which involved them in trying to pursue undeviatingly their chosen path through life. This corresponds to their wish – and consequent attempt – to keep driving straight on along their respective roads. Nevertheless, there are crossroads not only in the traffic context, but in life too. The straight road is the norm in life: it is that which one goes on pursuing out of sheer habit. The fact that all those involved suddenly found their straight-line progress interrupted by the accident shows that they had all failed to recognise the necessity for a change of course. Every direction and every norm in life eventually outlives its usefulness and creates the need for a change. In the course of time, everything that is right becomes wrong. People generally defend their norms with reference to the latter's past validity. But that is no argument. For a baby it is the norm to wet its nappies or diapers – and so it should be. But 5-year-old bed-wetters have no right to use this fact as a justification for their own symptom.

It is one of our more difficult challenges in life to recognise in good time the need for a change. This is something that those involved in our road-accident surely failed to recognise. They tried to pursue undeviatingly the course which they had quite justifiably been following thus far, while repressing the challenge to forsake the norm, to alter course, to get out of their current rut. Yet the impulse was still there unconsciously. Unconsciously, in other words, the path currently being followed was no longer appropriate. Yet they lacked the courage consciously to question it and so to abandon it. Change always arouses fear. 'We would really like to change' – but still we dare not. It could be a case of a partnership that has run its course, or of a job, or equally of a person's general outlook on life. Common to them all, however, is the repression of the desire to break free of old-established habit and custom. This unexpressed wish then seeks its realisation via some unconsciously willed event, which is always perceived by the conscious mind as coming from 'out there': those concerned are thrown off the road – in our example via the medium of a car-accident.

Those of us who are honest with ourselves are quite capable of recognising in the aftermath of such an event that, deep down inside, we had actually long since been discontent with the path that we were following and, though keen to abandon it, lacked the courage to do so. What happens to us is only ever what we *want* to happen. Unconscious solutions are admittedly quite successful, but they have the disadvantage that they are no real, ultimate answer to the problem. This is simply because any given problem can only be solved through a conscious step forward, whereas an unconscious solution does no more than represent its physical manifestation. That manifestation can provide an impulse. It can inform us too. But it cannot solve the problem totally.

Thus it is that, in our example, the car-accident frees those involved from their accustomed path, but at the same time restricts their freedom even more by trapping them inside the car. This new, unexpected situation is more than just an expression of the unconscious nature of what is going on; it can also be seen as a warning that leaving the accustomed road can lead not to the hoped-for freedom, but to a whole new form of imprisonment. The cries for help from the trapped and wounded were all but drowned by loud radio-music from inside the car. Those of us who are used to taking all events and manifestations as visible metaphors will equally see in this detail an expression of the occupants' attempt to divert their own attention from their inner conflict by means of mere externals. Radio-music is a way of drowning out the inner voice that is calling for help and is so anxious to be heard in its extremity by the conscious mind. But the conscious mind turns a deaf ear, refuses to listen, and so the conflict and the desire for freedom stay walled up in the unconscious. Neither can free itself by its own efforts: both have to wait for external events to set them free. In the current case the accident was the 'external event' that opened a channel for the unconscious problems to articulate themselves. The soul's cries for help became physically audible. Thus it is that human beings become honest.

Domestic and Occupational Accidents

Just as in the case of road-accidents, the number of possible symbolisms underlying the remaining types of accident at home and at work is almost unlimited, and therefore these need to be investigated individually and in detail.

We find, for example, a rich range of symbolism in connection with burns. A good many figures of speech use burning and fire as symbols for psychological processes: to 'burn one's tongue' – to 'burn one's fingers' – 'like grasping a red-hot poker' – to 'play with fire' – to 'go through fire and water' for someone.

Here 'fire' is more or less equivalent to 'danger'. Burns are thus signs that we have failed to assess the danger properly, or indeed have failed to spot them at all. Possibly we are failing to see what 'burning issues' are at stake. Burns make us aware of the fact that we are 'playing with fire'. What is more, fire also has a clear association with the subject of love and sexuality. Thus we speak of 'ardent (burning) love'. We may reach the point of being 'on fire with love' – at which point, naturally, we are 'aflame with desire'. We may even go on to refer to our lover as our 'flame'. Fire's sexual symbolism is even apparent in young people's love-relationships with their motorbikes: 'Let's go for a burn-up', they say, or 'I burned him off' (though here the fire is external rather than internal!).

Burns primarily affect the skin – which signifies people's limits. This compromising of our limits always indicates a calling into question of the ego. It is with our ego that we cut ourselves off from others, and this is precisely what gets in the way of love. In order to fall in love, we need to open up the limits of our ego; we have to catch fire, let love's embers set us alight and burn down all our barriers. Those who are not prepared to do so may well find that, in place of the inner fire, the outer barrier that is their skin is burnt by some external fire, so forcibly opening them up and making them vulnerable.

A similar symbolism is to be found in most other injuries that start by penetrating the outer barrier that is our skin. Moreover, we also speak of *psychological* wounds or traumas (Greek: 'wounds'); or again, we speak of people feeling 'wounded' by a remark. But of course it is possible not merely to wound others, but to 'cut off our nose to spite our face'. The symbolism underlying our 'falls' and 'stumblings' is every bit as transparent. A good many of us slip up on the ice because we 'haven't a leg to stand on'; others 'fall over their own feet', to say nothing of other people's. If concussion results, the subject's whole system of thought is fundamentally shaken up and compromised. Every attempt to sit up leads to headaches, with the result that he or she immediately lies down again. In this way both head and thought have their long-accustomed dominance automatically taken away from them, and patients learn from their own bodies that their thinking actually *hurts*.

Broken Bones

Almost without exception, bones break in situations of extreme mobility (whether car-crashes, motorbike-crashes or sporting clashes) as a direct result of external mechanical influences. The breakage leads straight to a longish period of enforced rest (whether in bed or in a plaster-cast). Every bone-fracture produces an *inter-ruption* of (a 'breakage between') our normal movement and activity, and makes us rest. Out of this enforced passivity and quietude some new attitude or orientation may well emerge. The fracture shows clearly that the growing need to bring some current development to an end has been ignored, so that the body itself is obliged to demonstrate the *breaking off* of the old in order to promote the *breakthrough* of the new. The breakage interrupts the former path, characterised as it was mainly by frenetic activity and movement. The patient has overdone and over-extended all the movement and stress; in other words he or she has generally 'screwed things up'.

Within the body, our bone represents the principle of firmness, of anchoring norms, but also of rigidity. If the rigidity-principle is over-predominant in the bone, it becomes brittle and for this reason can no longer fulfil its function. So it is, too, with our norms: while they provide us with points of anchorage, they can no longer do so if they become too rigid. A bone-fracture is a physical indication of a failure to notice that our psychological system is getting too rigid. In consequence we become too stiff, too unyielding and too inflexible. Just as there is a tendency for people to stand more and more on their basic principles as they grow older, in the process increasingly losing their psychological adaptability, so by the same token the calcification of the bones also builds up in time, with the result that the risk of fractures increases. The diametrical opposite of this situation is exemplified by the infant with its flexible and virtually unbreakable bones. The infant, after all, has as yet no norms or criteria to insist on. When we, on the other hand, become too inflexible in the way we live, a cracked vertebra will soon correct this lopsidedness – in fact it will literally 'break our back'. It is a fate that can be *de-flected* only by willingly becoming more *flex-ible*.

Thirteen

Psychological Symptoms

Under this heading we propose to deal with one or two common disorders that are normally classed as 'psychological'. At the same time it should be obvious how little sense such a description has in the context of our current approach. For in reality it is just not possible to draw a sharp dividing-line between somatic and psychological symptoms. Every symptom has a psychological content *and* expresses itself via the body. Even such conditions as anxiety or depression use the body as a tool for realising themselves. It is such somatic correlations that provide even academic psychiatric medicine with the basis for its pharmacological interventions. The tears of a depressive patient are no more 'psychological' than pus or diarrhoea. Such distinctions as there are seem to be most clearly justified at either end of the spectrum, where organic degeneration can be contrasted, for example, with a psychotic personality-change. But the further we move away from the two ends towards the centre-ground, the more difficult it becomes to find any clear dividing-line between the two. But then, on closer examination, even a consideration of the two extremes in no way justifies the distinction between 'somatic' and 'psychological', since that distinction depends purely on the type and form of symbolic expression involved. The symptomatology of asthma is just as different from an amputated leg as it is from schizophrenia. In short, the classification into 'somatic' and 'psychological' brings about more misunderstanding than clarity.

For our part, we in any case see no need for such distinctions, for our theory is universally applicable to all symptoms, and brooks no exceptions. Symptoms can admittedly employ a whole variety of forms for expressing themselves through, and yet to do so they all make use of the body for making the underlying contents of consciousness visible and tangible. At the same time, however, the actual experiencing of the symptom once again takes place exclusively within our consciousness – be it sadness or the pain of a wound. In Part 1 we pointed out that everything is a perfectly valid symptom in itself, and that it is only our own subjective evaluation that labels it either 'sick' or 'healthy'. Exactly the same thing applies in the so-called psychological sphere.

At this point we ought equally to free ourselves from the supposition that there are such things as 'normal' and 'abnormal' behaviour. 'Normality' is a statement of statistical frequency and therefore of no use either as a term of classification or as an evaluative yardstick. Granted, normality has the effect of reducing anxiety; but it also tends to work against individuation. Having to defend normality is one of the heaviest crosses that traditional psychiatry has to bear. A hallucination is neither more unreal nor more real than any other perception. It merely lacks the approval of the collective. Those who are 'psychologically ill' operate under exactly the same psychological laws as everybody else. Paranoiacs who imagine that they are being pursued and threatened by murderers project their own shadow on to those around them in exactly the same way as all those good, honest citizens who demand stronger punishments for offenders or live in constant fear of terrorists. Every projection is a delusion, and therefore the question as to when a delusion is 'normal' and when it is 'pathological' is in itself quite futile.

Psychological illness and psychological health are the theoretical end-points of a single continuum which arises out of the interplay between consciousness and the shadow. In so-called psychotics we find the result of successful repression in its most extreme form. Once all possible channels and contexts for living out the shadow are absolutely firmly closed, sooner or later there occurs a transfer of power, with the shadow taking over total control of the personality. In the process it suppresses – every bit as absolutely – that aspect of the consciousness which has hitherto been in control, and energetically makes up for everything that the patient's other aspect has hitherto lacked the confidence to live out. Thus it is that upright moralists turn into obscene exhibitionists, timid, gentle souls into wild, raging brutes, and diffident failures into megalomanics.

Psychosis too, then, makes us honest, in that it makes up for all our lost personal ground with an intensity and totality which those around us find frightening. It is a desperate attempt to bring all life's one-sidedness back into balance again – an attempt, however, which runs the risk of never again finding any way out of the constant alternation between extremes. Just how hard it is to discover the balanced, happy medium is particularly obvious in the case of the manic-depressive syndrome. Psychosis is a way of living out one's shadow. Madness has consequently always produced a mixture of fear and helplessness in its beholders, because it reminds them of their own shadows. Those who are mad effectively open up for us a door into the mental hell that lies deep within all of us. Thus, the anxious, feverish combating and suppression of this symptom is understandable enough, even if it is hardly suited to solving the problem. Indeed, the whole principle of suppressing the shadow can only lead directly to a violent explosion. Repeated suppression may put off the problem to another day, but ultimately it solves nothing and saves nobody.

The first essential step in the other direction is once again to recognise that the symptom is both meaningful and perfectly justified in its own right. Building on this insight, we can then start thinking about how best to help promote the symptom's health-giving aims.

These few observations on the subject of psychotic symptoms should suffice for the present. Detailed interpretations in this particular context do not get us very far, since psychotics are not in any case amenable to such interpretations. So great is their fear of their own shadow that they tend for the most part to project it exclusively outwards. Interested observers will, however, have little difficulty in arriving at an interpretation provided that they bear in mind the two rules that have already been mentioned repeatedly in this book, namely:

1.   Everything that is experienced by patients as an outward event is a projection of their own shadow (voices, attacks, persecutions, hypnotisers, murderous intentions and so on).
2.   Patients' psychological behaviour is itself a forcible manifestation of their neglected shadow.

But then, in the last event, psychological symptoms are not really susceptible of interpretation at all, since they are already expressing the problem directly and do not need to be translated onto any other level. For this reason anything one cares to say about the problems attending psychological symptoms soon starts to sound trite, since the translation stage is missing. Nevertheless we do propose in this context to discuss three symptoms by way of example, in the light of the fact that they have a wide distribution and are commonly allocated to the psychological sphere – namely depression, insomnia and addiction.

Depression

'Depression' is an umbrella-term for a symptomatic picture that ranges from a mere feeling of being 'down' and a general loss of motivation to so-called endogenous depression with its characteristic total apathy. Alongside a total block on all activity and the depressed mood itself, we also tend to encounter in depression a whole panoply of accompanying physical symptoms, foremost among which are tiredness, sleep-disorders, loss of appetite, constipation, headaches, heart-palpitations, lumbago, disturbed periods in women and loss of body-tone. Depressives are plagued with strong feelings of guilt and self-reproach, and constantly worry about making restitution. The word 'depression' derives from the Latin verb *deprimo*, which means 'to press down' or 'to press under'. This immediately raises the question of what it is that depressives feel that they are being pressed down by, or indeed what they themselves are *sup-pressing*. By way of an answer, we find ourselves confronted with three subject areas:

1. *Aggression*

We said earlier that aggression which finds no outlet transforms itself into bodily pain. This observation needs to be extended to include the fact that aggression that is suppressed at the psychological level leads to depression. Aggression whose expression is blocked gets turned inwards to the point where the transmitter becomes the receiver. The repressed aggression is responsible not only for the guilt-feelings, but also for the numerous accompanying symptoms, with their various types of pain. We have already pointed out elsewhere that aggression is merely a particular form of life-energy and activity. Thus, those of us who anxiously repress their aggressive impulses simultaneously repress all their energy and activity too. Eager though psychiatry is to involve depressives in some kind of activity again, the latter merely find this threatening. They compulsively avoid anything that fails to meet with general approval, and attempt to hush up their aggressive, destructive urges by living a life that is beyond reproach. Self-directed aggression finds its clearest expression in suicide. Suicidal tendencies should always prompt us to look into just who the murderous intentions are really aimed at.

2. Responsibility

Suicide apart, depression is the ultimate way of avoiding taking responsibility. Depressives no longer act, but simply vegetate, more dead than alive. Yet despite their constant refusal to get to active grips with life, depressives merely go on to find themselves confronted with the theme of responsibility via the back door of their own guilt-feelings. This fear of taking responsibility is well to the fore in those depressions that strike at the moment when patients are faced with embarking on some new phase of life, as is exemplified particularly clearly in the case of puerperal depression.

3. Withdrawal – loneliness – old age – death

These four closely related topics serve to sum up the final and (to our way of thinking) most important of our three subject areas. Depression has the effect of forcing patients to come to terms with life's mortal pole. Depressives are deprived of all that is truly alive, such as movement, change, companionship and communication, and in their place life's opposite pole manifests itself: apathy, rigidity, loneliness, thoughts of death. Indeed, this death-aspect of life which makes itself so vividly felt in depression is nothing more or less than the patient's own shadow.

The conflict then, lies in the fact that the depressed person is just as afraid of living as of dying. Active living inevitably brings with it guilt and responsibility – and it is these that the depressive is above all determined to avoid. Accepting responsibility also means abandoning all projections and accepting one's own *all-one-ness*. Depressive personalities, however, are afraid to do this, and therefore need other people to hang on to. Separation from such intimates can, like their death, quite often be the external trigger for depression. Those concerned, after all, are now left on their own – and living alone and taking responsibility are just what they least want to do. Being afraid of death, they fail to grasp life's conditionalities either. Depression makes us honest: it brings to light our incapacity both for living and for dying.

Insomnia

The number of people who suffer from more or less prolonged sleep disorders is very great. Equally great, consequently, is the consumption of sleeping-tablets. Just like eating and sex, sleep is a basic and instinctive human need. We spend a third of our lives in this state. A safe, secure and comfortable sleeping-place is of central significance for human and beast alike. Tired animals, like tired people, are quite prepared to cover large distances just in order to find somewhere suitable to sleep. We react with great irritation to having our sleep disturbed, and regard sleep-deprivation as one of the greatest threats to us. Having a good sleep is generally bound up with a whole range of familiar circumstances: a particular bed, a particular sleeping position, a particular time of day, and so on. Any disruption of these conditions is quite liable to disrupt our sleep too.

Sleep is a strange business. We all manage to sleep without ever having learnt to, and yet we have no idea how it works. We spend a third of our life in this particular state of consciousness, and yet know next to nothing about this whole area. We long for sleep – and yet we often feel threatened by the world of sleep and dreams. We are only too keen to ward off such incipient fears with comments such as 'It was only a dream,' or 'Dreaming is just seeming.' But if we are honest, we have to admit that our dreamworld seems just as real to us at the time as does our waking world during the day. Those of us who are prepared to meditate on this fact are perhaps best placed to appreciate the point that the world of our daytime consciousness is just as much an illusion, just as much a dream, as is our nightly dreamworld, and that both worlds exist only in our minds.

Whence, then, comes our belief that the life that we lead day by day is any more real or genuine than our dreamlife? What right do we have to qualify our dreams with the word 'only'? Every experience gained by our consciousness is equally real – regardless of whether we call it 'reality', 'dream' or 'fantasy'. It could thus be a useful mental exercise for us to reverse the ways in which we normally regard daytime happenings and dream-events, in such a way as to see dreaming as a continuous life-process that is interrupted on a regular basis by a 'sleeping' phase corresponding to our everyday life.

'Wang dreamed that he was a butterfly. He settled on the flowers among the grass. He fluttered hither and thither. Then he woke up, and could no longer tell whether he was Wang dreaming that he was a butterfly or a butterfly dreaming that it was Wang.'

Turning things upside-down in this way can be a good exercise for recognising that there is no obvious reason for assuming that either is any more real or actual than the other. Waking and sleeping, daytime and dreaming consciousness are mutually compensatory polarities. Analogically speaking, it is waking, living and activity that correspond to daytime and light, while it is darkness, inactivity, the unconscious and death that correspond to night.

Analogies

yang	yin
masculine	feminine
left brain	right brain
fire	water
day	night
waking	sleeping
life	death
good	evil
conscious	unconscious
intellect	feelings
rational	irrational

In line with this archetypal group of analogies, folk-tradition describes sleep as 'death's little brother'. Every time we go to sleep we are in fact practising dying. Falling asleep demands of us that we let go of all control, of all intentionality, of all active participation. It demands of us surrender and total trust, a letting-in of the unknown. In no way is it to be compelled by force, self-control, will or effort. The slightest act of will is the surest way of keeping sleep at bay. We can do no more than create the right conditions: then we simply have to wait patiently and trust that *it* will happen, that sleep will descend upon us. We are hardly given a chance even to observe the process – for the very observation itself would prevent us falling asleep.

What sleep (like death) demands of us, then, is not one of our strong points. We are too closely wedded to the active pole, too proud of our own deeds and achievements, too dependent on our intellect and our control over a reality that we basically mistrust for surrender, trust and letting go ever to become familiar forms of behaviour for us. Consequently nobody should be surprised at the fact that insomnia (along with headaches!) is reckoned to be among the most widespread disorders affecting the health of the civilised world.

Because of its one-sidedness, our culture has difficulty in coping with such alternative aspects of life, as is immediately apparent from the list of analogies tabulated above. We are afraid of our feelings, of the irrational, of our shadow, of the unconscious, of evil, of darkness and of death. We feverishly hang on to our intellect and our daytime consciousness, imagining that they will somehow reveal everything to us. When, consequently, the challenge comes to let go, fear strikes home, for the loss involved seems to us too great. And yet we long for sleep and are well aware of how much we need it. Just as night belongs to day, so our shadow belongs to our waking consciousness, and death to life. Sleep brings us daily to the threshold between the here and the beyond, leads us into our soul's own realm of night and shadow, allows us to live out in our dreams what we have failed to live out during the day, and so brings us back into balance.

Those of us who suffer from insomnia – or, to put it more accurately, from problems with going to sleep – are people who have difficulty in releasing their conscious grip and who are afraid of their own unconscious. Nowadays, after all, we hardly make any break between day and night, instead taking all our thoughts and activities over with us into the world of sleep. We prolong the day far into the night – in much the same way as we endeavour to analyse the night side of our soul using the techniques of our daytime consciousness. There is no break, no hiatus to act as a deliberate reversal or switchover point.

The first thing that insomniacs need to learn is to bring the day consciously to a close, so as to be able to give themselves over totally to the night and its laws. They further need to learn to engage their unconscious in an effort to find out what lies at the basis of their fear. Transitoriness and death are important issues for them. Insomniacs are lacking in native trust and the capacity for self-surrender. They identify too strongly with the 'doer' and never manage to let themselves go. The underlying themes here are almost identical to those that we noted in the case of orgasm. Sleep and orgasm are both 'little deaths' and are regarded as threatening by those with a strong ego-identification. It follows, then, that reconciliation with the night-side of life is a sure-fire soporific.

Old, familiar tricks such as counting sheep likewise owe such success as they have purely to the consequent letting go of the intellect. Anything monotonous simply 'bores the pants off'* the left half of the brain and causes it to let go of its dominance. All meditation techniques make use of this basic principle: concentrating on a single point or on the breath, repeating a

---

The very expression suggests a de-activation of the 'masculine', intellectual, conscious mind. – tr.

mantra or a *koan* – all of these lead to a switchover from left to right, from the day-side to the night-side, from activity to passivity. Those who find this natural rhythmic alternation difficult should get to grips with the particular pole that they are avoiding. Indeed, this is precisely what the symptom itself is trying to bring about. It gives those concerned a whole lot of time for coming to terms with night's fears and more sinister aspects. Once again, in other words, the symptom makes us honest: insomniacs are afraid of the night. Precisely so.

An exaggerated sleep-drive is a sign of the opposite problem. Those who despite sufficient sleep still have fundamental problems both with waking up and with getting up need to take a look at their fear of what the day demands – activity and work. Waking up and starting the day means becoming active, doing things and taking responsibility for them. Those who find the switch to day-consciousness too hard a step to take are taking refuge in the dreamworld and unconsciousness of childhood and ducking life's challenges and responsibilities. In such cases the name of the game is flight into the unconscious. Just as going to sleep is related to dying, so waking up is a little birth. Being born and becoming conscious can turn just as frightening as night and death. The problem, then, lies in one-sidedness. The solution lies in the happy medium, in balance, in both/and. Only at this point does it finally become apparent that birth and death are one.

SLEEP DISORDERS

Sleeplessness should be taken as a cue for asking the following:

1. How dependent am I on power, control, intellect and observation?
2. Am I able to let go?
3. How developed are my facility for self-surrender and my innate trust?
4. Am I having sufficient regard for the night-side of my soul?
5. How afraid am I of death? Have I come to terms with it sufficiently?

An exaggerated need for sleep throws up the questions:

1. Am I running away from activity, responsibility and consciousness-development?
2. Am I living in a dreamworld, afraid to wake up to reality?

Addictive Conditions

The subject of the exaggerated sleep-drive brings us directly to the various addictions, for here, too, running away from things is the central problem at issue. An addiction, after all, is a craving. Addicts are people who crave something, yet who have called off their search prematurely, getting themselves stuck on some kind of substitute level. Every search needs to lead to eventual discovery, and so to its own fulfilment. As Jesus said: 'He who seeks should not cease from seeking until he finds; and when he finds, he will be shaken; and when he has been shaken he will marvel and will reign over the All' (Gospel of Thomas, Log. 2).

All the great heroes of mythology and literature are engaged in searches or quests – Odysseus, Don Quixote, Parsifal, Faust – yet they do not cease searching until they have attained their goal. The quest leads the hero through danger, confusion, despair and darkness. Yet once they have found what they are looking for, what they discover makes all their efforts seem as nothing. We are all involved in some kind of odyssey, and in the course of it we are driven onto the strangest shores of the soul – yet we should never hang fire or allow ourselves to get bogged down, but should always keep searching until we find our goal.

'Seek, and you shall find,' says the gospel. But those who are scared off by the trials and dangers, the troubles and the confusions along the way merely turn into freaks, or addicts. They project the goal of their search onto something or other that they have already discovered along the way, and promptly call off their quest. They become besotted with this substitute goal and never tire of it. They attempt to satisfy their hunger with more and more of the self-same junk-food, not noticing that the more they eat the hungrier they get. They have thus become, *junkies*, or addicts, who refuse to admit that in fact they have mistaken their goal and need to go on looking. They are firmly in the grip of fear, indolence and delusion. Every stop along the way can turn us into such freaks. The sirens lurk everywhere, doing their utmost to hold wanderers fast and bind them to themselves – in other words, to turn them into addicts.

So long as we fail to see through it, absolutely anything in the world of forms can become addictive: money, power, fame, possessions, influence, knowledge, pleasure, eating, drinking, asceticism, religious ideas, drugs. All of them – whatever they are – are perfectly valid as experiences *per se*, yet at the same time anything at all can turn into an 'addictive substance' if we neglect to free ourselves again from its clutches. Addiction is cowardice in the face of new experiences. True seekers, as opposed to addicts, are people who view life as a journey and are always on the move. In order to know what it is like to be a seeker, we have to admit to being of no fixed abode. Those of us who believe in obligations, then, are addicted right from the start. All of us have our particular 'addictive substances' that cause us to turn a deaf psychological ear to what is really going on. The problem, though, is not so much the substances themselves as the lazy way in which we go about our search. At best, a consideration of our addictive substances reveals to us the main subjects of our `longing. It is all too easy to take an unbalanced view if we lose sight of those 'addictive substances' that are socially acceptable – riches, hard work, success, knowledge and so on. Bearing this in mind, however, the particular 'addictive substances' that we propose to consider briefly here are all ones that are commonly accepted as being pathological in character.

Compulsive eating

Living implies learning. Learning means integrating and incorporating into our consciousness principles which have hitherto been regarded as external to the 'I'. This constant absorption of the new leads to consciousness-expansion. It is possible, though, to replace 'spiritual nourishment' with physical nourishment, whose *in-corporation* merely leads to bodily expansion. If our hunger for life is not satisfied through actual experience, it is precipitated into the body, where it makes itself felt as plain hunger. But this is a hunger that cannot be appeased, for inner emptiness cannot be satisfied with physical food.

We said in an earlier chapter that love is really self-opening and acceptance. Compulsive eaters, however, live out their love only via the body, being unable to manage it at the level of consciousness. They long for love, but instead of opening up the boundaries of their ego, they merely open up their mouths and gobble up everything in sight. The result is sometimes referred to as 'worry-fat'. Compulsive eaters are in search of love, of approval, of reward – but unfortunately on the wrong level.

Alcohol

Alcoholics are people who are longing for an ideal, conflict-free world. There is nothing wrong with that aim, except that they try to achieve it by avoiding their conflicts and problems, using alcohol to give them the illusion that everything in the garden is lovely. Most alcoholics also seek out close human company. The alcohol creates a kind of caricature of human closeness by dismantling restrictions and inhibitions, blurring social distinctions and speeding up the process of making friends – though in the absence of any real depth or intimacy. Alcohol is an attempt to fulfil the quest for an ideal, conflict-free world of universal brotherhood. Anything that stands in the way of this ideal has to be drowned out in the shortest possible order.

Cigarettes

Smoking's main link is with the body's airways and lungs. We should recall that breathing is mainly concerned with communication, contact and freedom. Smoking is an attempt to stimulate and satisfy these areas. Cigarettes are turned into substitutes for real communication and freedom. Cigarette-advertising is deliberately aimed at such human longings: the freedom of the cowboy, aviation's transcendence of all barriers, journeys to distant lands and the companionship of happy people – all these longings on the part of the ego are, it seems, to be satisfied with a cigarette. We travel for miles, and why? For a woman, for a friend, or perhaps just to be free. Or else ... we substitute a cigarette for all these genuine desires, and the cigarette-smoke veils our real goal.

Drugs

The theme behind hashish (marihuana) is extremely similar to that underlying alcohol. Drug-addicts use the cosiness of the drug-state to escape their problems and conflicts. Hashish takes away all life's hardness and sharp edges. Everything becomes softer and life's challenges fade into the background.

Cocaine (like similar stimulants such as Captagon) has the opposite effect. It improves its users' performance enormously and in this way can to some extent lead to greater success. At this point, therefore, the theme of success, performance and recognition needs to be looked into, since the drug is merely a means of dramatically improving one's performance. The search for success is always a search for love. It is for this reason that in show-business and the film-world, for example, cocaine is particularly widely used. The hunger for love is show-business's specific occupational problem. The artists who put themselves on show are longing for love and hoping to satisfy this longing with public acclaim. (The fact that this is not actually possible does tend on the one hand to improve their performance, but on the other hand it also makes them psychologically more and more unhappy!) With or without the presence of stimulant drugs, the addictive substance here is actually *success*, whose role is to replace the actual search for love.

As for heroin, this makes it possible for the addict to run away utterly and totally from coming to grips with the world as it is.

The psychedelic drugs (LSD, mescalin, 'magic mushrooms' and so on) are very clearly delineated from the drugs mentioned so far. Behind the taking of these mind-blowing drugs lies the intention (more or less conscious) to seek new psychological experiences and enter the world of the transcendent. In the narrower sense, moreover, psychedelic drugs are not addictive. Whether they represent legitimate tools for opening up new dimensions of consciousness is not easy to decide, since the problem does not lie in the drugs themselves, but in the consciousness of those who use them. The only thing that can ever be ours is what we ourselves have wrought. For this reason it is generally extremely difficult to make the new areas of consciousness opened up by drugs truly our own without being overwhelmed by them. The further we go along this road, the more dangerous the drugs become for us – but then the less we need them, too. Everything that can be achieved with the aid of drugs can be achieved without them – only more slowly. And haste is itself a dangerous addictive substance along our way!

Fourteen

Cancer

If we are to understand cancer, it is particularly important for us to think in analogical terms. We need to make ourselves fully alive to the fact that every whole entity that we perceive or define (every whole among other wholes) on the one hand is part of a greater whole, and on the other hand is simultaneously composed of many lesser wholes. Thus a wood, for example, is (as a defined whole) not only a part of the greater whole that is the countryside, but is itself composed of many trees (smaller wholes). The same goes in turn for each individual tree. Not only is it a part of the wood, but it also consists of a trunk, roots and crown. The trunk's relationship to the tree is the same as that of the tree to the wood or of the wood to the countryside generally.

Each of us is a part of humanity, while ourselves consisting of organs that not only are parts of a human being, but at the same time are made up of a multiplicity of cells that in their turn are parts of the organ itself. Humanity expects each of us as individual human beings to do our best to behave in such a way as best serves the development and survival of humanity as a whole. Each of us in turn expects our organs to work in the best interests of our survival as human beings. And the organ expects its own cells to fulfil their duty in respect of the organ's own survival.

Within this hierarchy, which can be extended *ad infinitum* in both directions, each individual whole (be it cell, organ or human being) is in a situation of constant conflict between its own particular life on the one hand and subordination to the interests of the next entity up the scale on the other. Each complex organism (humanity, state, organ) has its functioning ordered in such a way that as far as possible all its parts defer to the one common idea and work on its behalf. Each system can normally cope with the failure of a few of its constituent parts without any danger to the whole. Yet there is a limit beyond which the very existence of the whole is put at risk.

Thus, a state can cope with some of its citizens refusing to work, behaving antisocially or setting themselves up against the state. If, however, this group of *refuseniks* increases in numbers, it can eventually reach a size where it starts to become a serious danger to the whole: indeed, should it turn into a majority it can threaten the whole's continued existence. Naturally the state will devote much time to trying to protect itself against this development and fighting for its own existence, but should it fail in the attempt its collapse is inevitable. The most promising available approach would be to bring the dissidents back into the fold in good time, while they are still at the small-group stage, by offering them attractive opportunities to co-operate in working towards the common goal. In the long run, though, the method usually applied by the state is violently to suppress or eradicate the disaffected elements – and this is hardly ever successful: indeed, this reaction is more likely to lead to chaos. From the state's point of view the forces of opposition are dangerous enemies whose sole aim is to destroy the 'good old order' and spread chaos abroad.

This way of looking at things is perfectly justified, of course – though only from one particular viewpoint. Were we to ask those rebelling against the established order for their opinions, we should hear other arguments that would be equally justified – from *their* point of view, that is. Obviously, though, they would not be identifying themselves with the state's aims and ideas, but setting up in opposition to them views and interests of their own which *they* would be keen to see put into effect. What the state wants is obedience: what such groups want, by contrast, is freedom to realise their own ideas. We can well understand both sides, but it is not easy to realise both sets of interests at once without making certain sacrifices.

In no way is it the purpose of these few lines to develop any kind of political or social theory or creed: rather is it to represent what happens in cancer in a different context, so as to broaden somewhat people's normally extremely blinkered view of the disease. Cancer is not an isolated occurrence whose sole manifestation is the illness that is so called: rather are we confronted in cancer with a very sophisticated and intelligent process which is of equal concern to us on every other level, too. In virtually every other illness we find the body trying to get rid of whatever problem is jeopardising its functions by applying suitable counter-measures. If it succeeds in this, we speak of 'healing' (which can be either more or less total). If it fails and goes under in the attempt, we call the result 'death'.

In the cancer-process, however, we are faced with something fundamentally different: the body merely looks on, as more and more of its own cells change their behaviour and begin a process of regular division which has no end in itself, but merely finds its ultimate term in the exhaustion of the host that is its food-source. The cancer-cell is not some external threat to the organism in the way that bacteria, viruses or toxins are, for example: instead, it is a cell that has hitherto devoted all its activity to the service of the organ in question, and thus to that of the organism as a whole, so as best to promote its prospects of survival. Yet suddenly it 'changes its mind' and abandons the common identification. It starts to develop its own aims and to put them into effect regardless of anything else. It ceases to perform what hitherto has been a specific organic role, and makes its own reproduction its first and only priority. It no longer behaves as a member of a multicellular life-form, but regresses to an evolutionarily more primitive form of existence as a single-celled organism. It terminates its membership of the Union of Cellular Workers and, thanks to its chaotic process of cell-division, goes on to spread itself abroad with great rapidity and ruthlessness, ignoring all morphological boundaries (infiltration) and establishing footholds all over the body (metastasis-formation). It uses what is left of the community from which its behaviour has expelled it as a host for feeding on. The cancer-cells grow and multiply so quickly that the blood-vessels are unable to maintain an adequate blood-supply. And so the cancer-cells switch from oxygen-breathing to the more primitive process of fermentation. Breathing is dependent on community (on exchange): fermentation is something that any cell can do for itself.

This highly successful process of self-dissemination on the part of the cancer-cells finally comes to a stop only when they have literally eaten up the person that they have used as their food-source. The cancer-cells eventually come to grief, in other words, over problems of supply. Right up until that moment their behaviour is perfectly successful.

There remains the question of why the formerly well-behaved cell should do all this. In fact its motivation should be quite easy to follow. As a dutiful constituent member of a multicellular human being, it merely had to perform the job laid down for it, which served to ensure the larger organism's survival. It was one cell among many, obliged to do an unattractive job for 'another'. And for a long time that was precisely what it did. At some point, however, the larger organism lost its attraction as a context for the cell's own development. A single-celled organism is free and independent, can do as it likes, can make itself immortal by propagating itself *ad infinitum*. As part of a multicellular organism the cell was both mortal and restricted. Is it so very astonishing, then, that the cell should recall its former freedom and revert to life as a single cell so as to realise its immortality by its own unaided efforts? It subordinates the former community of cells to its own interests and by its irresponsible behaviour starts to realise its own freedom.

A successful enough approach, certainly, whose basic flaw only becomes apparent later – namely when it becomes clear that sacrificing others and using them as a food-source necessarily brings with it the cell's own demise. Cancer-cells' behaviour is only successful so long as the human host survives: the latter's end also spells the end of the cancerous development itself.

At this point, then, we run into the small, but highly significant flaw in the whole idea of attaining freedom and immortality. To declare independence from the former community is also to realise – too late – how necessary it really was. Human beings are not at all happy to give up their lives for the sake of that of the cancer-cell; but then neither is the cancer-cell particularly happy to give up its own life for the human being of which it is part. The cancer-cell has just as good arguments on its side as the human being: it is just that its viewpoint is different. Both want to stay alive and to realise their own interests and their ideas of freedom. Both are quite prepared to sacrifice the other in the process. The same applies, too, where state politics are concerned, as in our earlier example. The state is anxious to stay alive and to put its ideas into effect; but the dissenting minority also want to stay alive and put *their* ideas into effect. To start with, consequently, the state does its utmost to victimise the 'awkward brigade'. If they fail, though, it is the revolutionaries who sacrifice the state instead. Neither party has the slightest regard for the other. Similarly, then, we operate on the cancer-cells and irradiate and poison them for as long as we can – but if they still win, it is we who are sacrificed. It is nature's age-old conflict: to eat or be eaten. Given, then, that we are aware of the cancer-cell's recklessness and short-sightedness, how far are we also aware that we ourselves behave in exactly the same way, trying to assure our own survival on the basis of the same cancerous concept?

This is where the key to the whole cancer-process lies. It is no accident that we today are so afflicted with cancer, so anxious to fight it and yet so unsuccessful in our attempts. (Investigations by the American cancer-researcher Hardin B. Jones have shown that the life-expectancy of untreated cancer-patients is apparently greater than that of treated ones!) As an illness, cancer is an expression of our time and of our collective outlook. What we undergo inwardly as cancer is merely what we ourselves are doing in our own lives. Our times are characterised by the reckless expansion and promotion of our own interests. In our political, economic, 'religious' and private life we do our ruthless utmost to push our own aims and interests to the ('morphological') limit; to establish bases for our interests here, there and everywhere (metastases); and to act as though only our own ideas and aims counted, while manipulating everybody else to our own advantage (parasitism).

Our whole rationale is just like that of the cancer-cell. So rapid and successful is our expansion that we, too, can barely cope with our supply-problems. Our communications-systems extend world-wide, yet still we cannot communicate with our neighbours or partners. We have leisure, yet we do not know what to do with it. We produce and destroy foodstuffs purely in order to manipulate prices. We can travel the whole world, yet still do not know ourselves. Our current philosophy knows no other goal but growth and progress. We work, experiment, research – yet for what? For the sake of progress! And what is the aim of that progress? Yet more progress! Humanity is on a trip without a goal. And so it constantly has to set itself new targets to keep despair at bay. The cancer-cell simply cannot hold a candle to the blindness and short-sightedness of contemporary humanity. For the sake of pursuing economic expansion, we have for decades been exploiting our environment as both larder and host, only to be 'astonished' by the sudden realisation that the death of the host also involves the death of humanity itself. We regard the whole world as a quarry to be mined – whether for plants, animals or raw-materials. The one and only reason why it is all there, it seems, is so that we can spread ourselves across the face of the earth *ad infinitum*.

In the light of this behaviour, how can we possibly have the gall or the sheer, bare-faced cheek to complain about cancer? All it is doing, after all, is mirroring what we ourselves get up to – our behaviour, our reasoning and even where it will all ultimately get us.

It is not a question of *conquering* cancer: it is merely a

question of understanding it, so that we can then learn to understand ourselves too. How keen we are to smash the mirror whenever we do not like the look of our face! If we become cancerous, it is because we *are* cancerous.

Cancer gives us our great opportunity to discover in it the extent of our own misunderstanding and false reasoning. Let us therefore do our best to discover the conceptual weak-points in the outlook that we and cancer have in common. Ultimately, cancer's great stumbling-block is the polarisation between 'me' and 'the community'. This 'either/or' is all it can see, and so it plumps for survival on its own account, independently of its environment – only to realise, too late, that it is actually *dependent* on that environment. It lacks any awareness of the larger, all-embracing unity. It sees unity only in terms of its own self-delineation. It is this misunderstanding of unity that we human beings share with cancer. We, too, divide ourselves off mentally, so giving rise to the split between 'I' and 'you'. We think in terms of 'unities' – or rather of 'units' – without realising the meaninglessness of such terms. Unity – oneness – is the sum of all being, outside of which there is nothing. Cut up unity into bits, and you get diversity – yet this diversity still ultimately adds up to unity.

The more the ego divides itself off, the more it loses the sense of that whole of which it is still a part. There arises in the ego the illusion that it can act 'alone'. Yet the word 'alone' literally means 'all-one' (that is, 'one with all'), and *not* total differentiation from everything else. For in reality there can be no real state of separation from the rest of the universe. It is something that exists only in our ego's imagination. To the extent that the 'I' boxes itself in, we lose our *religio*, our link with the original source of all being. At this point, then, the ego starts trying to satisfy its own needs, and dictates what path we are to follow. For the 'I', everything that serves to delimit and differentiate it yet further is all to the good, for every re-emphasis of its boundaries gives it a still clearer sense of itself. The only thing that the ego is afraid of is becoming 'all-one', for this would imply its own death. At great cost, therefore, and with much intelligence and a plethora of good arguments, the ego defends its own existence, commandeering the most sacrosanct of theories and the most noble of intentions to that end. Its sole aim is to survive.

So it is, then, that goals arise which are in fact nothing of the kind. As a goal, after all, progress itself is absurd, for it has no end-point. A genuine goal has to involve a change in the existing circumstances: it cannot imply a mere continuation of whatever is there already. As human beings, we are enmeshed in polarity: what, then, can we possibly hope to achieve by setting ourselves purely polar goals? If, on the other hand, our goal is oneness, then this implies a totally different quality of being from that which we experience in the polar context. To offer a person in prison the prospect of another prison is not something that is particularly attractive, even if it is a bit more comfortable – but to grant them their freedom is qualitatively a much more substantial step. Yet the goal of oneness can only be attained by giving up the 'I', for as long as there is an 'I' there is a 'you' as well – and just so long, consequently, we remain enmeshed in our polar world. The 'rebirth in the spirit' always presupposes a death, and this death is that of the ego. The Islamic mystic Rumi sums up this theme superbly in the following short story:

A man came to the door of the Beloved and knocked. A voice asked, 'Who is there?'
'It is I,' he replied.
Said the voice, 'There is not enough room here for me and thee.' And the door remained shut.
After a year of loneliness and privation the man came back and knocked again. From inside a voice asked, 'Who is there?'
'It is thou,' said the man. And the door was opened to him.

So long as our 'I' strives for eternal life, we shall fail in exactly the same way as the cancer-cell fails. What distinguishes the cancer-cell from the normal body-cell is an overestimation of its own ego. Within the cell, the nucleus corresponds to the cell's brain. In cancer-cells the nucleus continually gains in significance and thus also in size (cancer can even be diagnosed by morphological changes in the cell-nucleus). This change in the nucleus corresponds to an overemphasis on egocentric, cerebral thought, such as indeed characterises our own time. The cancer-cell seeks its eternal life through physical self-propagation and expansion. Neither cancer nor we ourselves have yet managed to grasp the fact that we are looking within physicality for something which is not to be found there, namely life itself. We confuse form with content, and endeavour to attain the content that we so long for through mere, formal reduplication. Jesus, though, long ago taught that 'he who would keep his life must lose it.'

Since the earliest times, therefore, every school of initiation has taught the opposite path; the once-and-for-all sacrifice of the formal aspect for the sake of attaining the content. In other words, the 'I' must die if we are ever to be reborn into the self. Note, though, that *self* does not mean *my*self, but *the* self. It is the centre that is everywhere. The self has no separate existence, for it embraces everything there is. At this point, then, the question 'I, or other people?' finally falls away. The self knows no 'others', for it is both 'alone' and 'all-one'. For the ego, such a goal naturally seems dangerous and unattractive. We have no right to be at all surprised, therefore, that the 'I' should prefer to trade in this goal of 'at-one-ment' for that of a big, strong, wise, enlightened ego. In pursuing the esoteric, no less than the religious path, most pilgrims' efforts founder precisely on the fact that they *will* endeavour to attain the goal of salvation or enlightenment *with their egos*. There are only very few who take the slightest account of the fact that the 'I' with which they persist in identifying themselves is by its very nature incapable of ever being saved or enlightened.

The Great Work, then, always involves the sacrifice of the 'I', the death of the ego. We cannot redeem our ego: all we can do is redeem ourselves *from* our ego – then indeed we are truly redeemed. Most of our fear of ceasing to exist that crops up at this point merely confirms how much we identify ourselves with our ego and how little we know about our true self. Yet, as far as our cancer-problem is concerned, this is actually where the possibility of salvation lies. Only as we learn slowly and gradually to put paid to our ego-based rigidity and self-delimitation – only, in short, as we learn to open ourselves up – can we start to feel part of the whole and thus also to take responsibility for the whole. At this point, too, we finally realise that the good of the whole and our own interests are one and the same – since we, as parts, are at the same time one with all (*pars pro toto*). Thus, every cell contains the whole of the organism's genetic information: surely, then, it can hardly help but realise that it is indeed the whole! As hermetic philosophy teaches us, 'Microcosmos = macrocosmos.'

The conceptual error lies in the differentiation of 'I' from 'you'. From this arises the illusion that we can promote our own survival specifically by exploiting and sacrificing the 'you'. In reality, however, the destiny of 'I' and 'you', of part and whole, is indivisible. The death in which the cancer-cell lands the organism as a whole turns out to be its own death, too, just as the death of our environment, for example, also spells out the death of humanity itself. Yet the cancer-cell persists in believing in a separate outer world, just as we do. This belief is fatal. And the only remedy is love. Love heals, because it opens up the barriers and lets in the Other with a view to becoming one with it. Those who are in love do not put their 'I' first, but experience a greater wholeness: they feel as though they themselves *were* their lovers. Nor does this only happen in the human context. There is no way in which anybody who loves an animal can take the farmer's view and regard it as a mere source of food. And we are not talking here of mere, sentimental pseudo-love, but of that state of consciousness which really senses something of the community of all existence. This is a far cry from the common attitude which results in people trying to compensate for their unconscious guilt-feelings about their own repressed aggressive urges with 'good works' or an exaggerated 'love of animals'. Cancer is a sign of unexpressed love – indeed, it is a perverted form of love.

Love transcends all bounds and barriers.

In love, the opposites unite and fuse together.

Love is union with all; it extends to everything and shrinks at nothing.

Love has no fear even of death – for love is life.

Those who fail consciously to live out this love run the risk that their love will descend into the body, where it will seek to realise its inner laws in the form of cancer.

Thus, cancer-cells, too, transcend all bounds and barriers: cancer, after all, dissolves the various organs' individualities.

Cancer, too, extends to everything and shrinks at nothing (metastasis).

Cancer-cells, too, have no fear of death.

Cancer is love at the wrong level. Total union is something that can be realised only at the level of consciousness, not within matter, for matter is consciousness's shadow. Within the context of the transitory world of forms we cannot achieve what properly belongs to the eternal level. Despite all the efforts of those who would improve the world, there will never be a perfect world without conflicts or problems, friction or confrontation. Neither will there ever be a healthy humanity without illness or death; nor, for that matter, all-embracing love, for the world of forms depends on boundaries. Yet all these goals can be attained – by anybody and at any time – by seeing through the forms and so achieving freedom at the level of consciousness. In the polar world, love leads to clinging: within unity it leads to pure outpouring and irradiation.* Cancer is the symptom of misunderstood love. Cancer treats true love only with respect. The symbol of true love is the heart. The heart is the only organ that cannot be attacked by cancer!

It is a striking reflection of this thought that irradiation is nowadays one of the conventionally approved forms of cancer-treatment – almost as though the latter were the 'shadow' of the true (and neglected) inner process, as indeed one might expect it to be. – tr.

Fifteen

AIDS

Since this book first appeared in Germany in 1983 a new disease has moved with a vengeance into the spotlight of public concern, and seems likely – as various indicators suggést – to stay there for a good long time. This new epidemic is symbolised by the four letters 'A.I.D.S.' – an abbreviation for 'Acquired Immune Deficiency Syndrome'. Its physical source is the HIV virus, a minute, highly sensitive disease-agent that is capable of surviving only in a very specific environment – which is why it is necessary for fresh blood-cells or sperm to enter the bloodstream of another person if the virus is to be transmitted to them. Outside the human organism the virus dies.

The natural reservoir of the AIDS virus is assumed to be certain species of monkey in Central Africa (notably the African green monkey). The virus was first discovered at the end of the 1970s in a New York drug-addict. Thanks to the sharing of hypodermic needles, the virus spread first among drug-addicts and from there into the homosexual community, where it was transmitted further through sexual contact. To this day it is homosexuals who are highest among the groups at risk, apparently because the anal intercourse favoured by them very often leads to damage to the sensitive mucous membrane of the anal passage, or rectum. This allows virus-carrying sperm to reach the bloodstream (the mucous membrane of the vagina, by contrast, is much less susceptible to injury).

AIDS first put in its appearance at precisely the moment when homosexuals in America had just managed considerably to improve and legitimise their social status. Since then it has in fact become known that in Central Africa AIDS is just as prevalent among heterosexuals. Nevertheless in America and Europe it is the homosexual community that has provided the seedbed for the epidemic. In the process all the sexual freedom and permissiveness achieved in our time has come under direct threat from the AIDS 'sex-plague'. Some regret the fact, while others see in it a piece of richly deserved divine retribution.

What is certain is that, as a result, AIDS has become a collective problem – for AIDS does not merely concern individuals, it concerns us all. That is why it seems sensible not only to us as authors, but also to our publisher, that we should include this additional chapter on AIDS, in which we should like to try and throw some light on its inherent symptomatology.

At the very outset of our consideration of the symptomatology of AIDS, four points particularly spring to mind:

1.   AIDS leads to the collapse of the body's own powers of resistance. That is, it weakens the body's ability to shut itself off from external disease-agents and to defend itself from them. This irreparable weakening of the immune-system's defences makes AIDS-sufferers susceptible to infections (as well as to various cancers) which pose no danger to healthy people whose defences are intact.

2.   Because the HIV virus has a very long incubation-period – several years can in fact elapse between the time of infection and the actual onset of illness – AIDS seems to have something particularly sinister about it. Other than by testing for antibodies to the AIDS virus (the Elisa method), one cannot tell how many people are infected overall, or whether one personally has the AIDS virus. In this way AIDS becomes an 'invisible opponent' which is consequently difficult to combat.

3.   Thanks to the fact that one can only catch AIDS by direct transmission, and that this in turn is directly bound up with blood and sperm, AIDS cannot remain a private or personal problem, but reminds us forcibly of our dependence on each other.

4.   Finally it remains for us to identify the principal theme of AIDS – namely sexuality, to which transmission is largely restricted (apart, that is, from the other two possibilities – injection with used hypodermic needles and transmission via blood-transfusions – both of which are relatively easy to eliminate as sources of risk). It is as a result of this fact that AIDS has acquired its status as a venereal disease, and that sexuality itself is now overshadowed by mortal fear.

The authors have become convinced that, as a collective disease-risk, AIDS is a natural extension of the problem that also manifests itself in cancer. Inherently, cancer and AIDS have a good deal in common, which is why both could be summed up under the heading 'love grown sick'. In order fully to understand what we mean by this, it is clearly fitting for us to go briefly once again into the theme of love, by way of recalling to mind what we said about it earlier. In Chapter 4 we learnt to see love as that condition which alone is capable of *over-coming* polarity and uniting the opposites. But since opposites are always defined by boundaries – between good and evil, inner and outer, I and you – love has the function of overcoming or (more accurately) of destroying those boundaries. Thus, love may be defined as the ability to open oneself up, to let in the 'other', to sacrifice the frontiers of the *I*.

The tradition of love-based sacrifice is a long and rich one in poetry, myth and religion alike: our own culture recognises it in the image of Jesus, who for love of humanity took upon himself the role of sacrificial victim and thus went the way of all sons of God. When we speak here of love, though, what we mean is a spiritual process, not a physical act: whenever we refer to 'physical love' we shall be employing explicitly sexual terms.

Once we are aware of this distinction, it must very quickly become obvious to us that our times and culture have a major problem where love is concerned. Love's prime focus is the other person's soul, not their body: it is *sexuality* that desires the other's body. Both, of course, have their *raison d'être*: the only danger lies – as ever – in one-sidedness. Life means balance, an equilibrium between yin and yang, between below and above, between left and right.

What this means in the context of our subject, then, is that sexuality has to be balanced out by love if we are not to finish up lopsided; and all lopsidedness is 'evil' – that is, *un-whole-some*, and thus sick. We are scarcely conscious any more of the vast overemphasis which our age places on the power of the ego and thus on self-delimitation, for this form of individualisation has by now become a matter of course for us. We have only to call to mind the importance nowadays accorded to proper names in industry, advertising and the arts, and to compare this with what used to happen in antiquity, when most artists remained totally anonymous, to become quite clear about what is meant here by an emphasis on the ego. This development is apparent in other areas of life, too – as, for example, in the change from the extended to the nuclear family, or to the unattached life-style that is currently so popular. The flat or apartment is a form of accommodation that is similarly an outward expression of our growing alienation and isolation.

Modern people do their best to counter this clear trend with two tools in particular – namely communications and sexuality. The development of the communications media is virtually falling over itself in its haste. What with newspapers, radio, television, telephones, computers, fax machines and so on, we are all becoming wired up and networked to each other. Yet, on the purely superficial level, electronic communications are too formal and non-committal to solve the problem of isolation and alienation, while at a deeper level the development of modern electronic systems makes it perfectly obvious to us how sense-less – indeed, impossible – it is to divide ourselves off from each other, to keep things secret from each other or to pursue ends that are purely egotistical in nature. (Secrecy, data-protection and copyright become all the more difficult and pointless the further the electronic revolution progresses!)

The second magic formula is 'sexual freedom': everybody is not only able, but willing, to contact and 'get in touch with' each other – while staying quite *un*touched at the spiritual level. It is thus no surprise to find the new communications media being placed at the service of sexuality, from the personal columns of the newspapers to telephone sex and computer sex (the latest game in the USA). In this way sexuality is put purely at the disposal of the satisfaction of personal desires – primarily one's own – with the 'partner' reduced to a mere tool. Ultimately, indeed, even the partner becomes unnecessary, for lust can have its way not only via the telephone, but in total isolation (masturbation).

Love, on the other hand, involves an honest encounter with another person. But then encountering 'the other' is always an anxious process, in that it involves throwing one's own 'such-ness' into question. An encounter with another person is always an encounter with one's own shadow, too. It is precisely because the latter is the way it is that partnership is so difficult. Love has more to do with work than with self-gratification. Love threatens the boundaries of our ego and demands that we open ourselves up. Sexuality is a marvellous aid to love, and on the bodily level it is also a splendid tool for overcoming the barriers and experiencing unity. But if we avoid love and merely experience sexuality, sex alone is incapable of fulfilling this task.

Our age, as we have said already, is ego-ridden to the nth degree, and strongly rejects anything that has as its goal the overcoming of polarity. Thus it is that we frantically attempt to conceal and make up for our unwillingness to love by laying great stress on sexuality. Our times are sexualised, yet loveless. Love falls into the shadows. The problem we have sketched out applies to our age and to our whole Western culture: it is a collective problem.

This problem, meanwhile, has crystallised in a particular way among homosexuals. We are not concerned here with the difference between homosexuality and heterosexuality, but with one pronounced development within the homosexual scene – namely a tendency to turn more and more away from a lasting relationship with a single partner towards promiscuity, with contact with ten or twenty partners in a single weekend being nothing out of the ordinary. Granted, this development and the problems that go with it apply just as much to heterosexuals as to homosexuals, yet this development has gone much further and become more extreme among homosexuals than within the heterosexual community.

The more love becomes divorced from sexuality, with sex merely a matter of physical self-gratification, the faster do the delights of sex tend to pall. This leads to a never-ending escalation of stimulation-levels: the triggering stimuli have to become ever more original, eccentric and ingenious in order to excite at all. This in turn results in very extreme sexual practices whose characteristics reveal quite clearly how little the other person has to do with it any more, and how much he or she has become degraded in the process into a mere object of stimulation.

This albeit sketchy account, we suggest, will suffice to enable us to understand the symptomatology of AIDS.

If love – in the sense of a spiritual meeting and encounter with another person – is no longer being lived out consciously, then it falls into the shadows and, in the last resort, descends into the body. Love is the principle of the undermining of barriers and of self-opening to incoming entities so as to become one with them. The collapse of the body's powers of resistance that occurs with AIDS corresponds exactly to this principle. It is precisely the job of the body's immune-system to defend its boundaries, which are of course essential for any life-form, since any such form predicates delimitation (and thus ego). The AIDS patient is living out on the bodily level the love, the openness and the associated accessibility and vulnerability which he or she is afraid to live out on the psychological level.

The theme underlying AIDS is very similar to that underlying cancer – which is why we have grouped both sets of symptoms under the heading of 'love grown sick'. But there is also a difference, in that cancer is more 'private' than AIDS – by which we mean that cancer affects patients much more as isolated individuals, and that it is not catching. AIDS, on the other hand, makes us ultra-aware that we are not alone in the world, that any kind of isolation is an illusion, and that the ego, in the last resort, is a mere mirage. AIDS makes us alive to the fact that we are for ever part of a community, part of a greater whole and are thus, as part, also responsible for all. All of a sudden the AIDS patient feels the enormous impact of this responsibility and from that moment on has to decide how to respond to it. AIDS ultimately forces us to take responsibility for others and to exercise care and consideration for them – themes which have hitherto figured too lightly in the lives of AIDS patients in particular.

Furthermore, AIDS forces upon us a total avoidance of sexual aggressiveness, for as soon as blood starts to flow the partner becomes contaminated. Through the use of condoms (and rubber gloves) the barriers that AIDS has contrived to take down on the bodily level are now built up again. In turning away from aggressive sex, patients have the chance to learn tenderness and gentleness as modes of encounter, while being brought by AIDS into contact with the long-avoided themes of weakness, powerlessness and passivity – in short, with the world of their feelings.

It rapidly becomes evident, then, that all those areas that AIDS forces into the background (aggression, blood, inconsideration...) reside within the masculine aspect of polarity (yang), whereas those themes which AIDS actually imposes on us (weakness, powerlessness, tenderness, gentleness, consideration...) belong to the feminine side of polarity (yin). It is no surprise, consequently, that AIDS should be so prominent among homosexuals, for the male *homo-sexual* ('same-sex-ish') is by definition avoiding the encounter with the feminine. (The fact that, even so, homosexual men themselves demonstrate strong feminine traits in their behaviour in no way contradicts the point, for these traits are themselves symptomatic of the case!)

The groups most at risk from AIDS are drug-addicts and homosexuals. These two groups are relatively sharply marked out from society at large. They are groups which the rest of society frequently spurns or even hates – groups, indeed, that even go out of their way to attract such rejection and hatred. What the body is living out and learning by falling prey to AIDS is the opposite of hate – the abandonment of all defences and thus love of all.

AIDS confronts humanity with a deeply buried region of the shadow. It is a messenger from the 'underworld' – and this in a double sense, for the disease-agents similarly gain entry via the human body's own 'underworld'. The virus itself spends a long time 'in the dark', unknown and unrecognised, until it slowly and insidiously penetrates the patient's awareness via increased physical susceptibility and degeneration. At this point AIDS demands a complete turnabout, a metamorphosis. AIDS seems sinister to us because it operates out of that which is hidden, unseen, unknown: it is the 'invisible opponent' by whom Amfortas the grail-king is incurably wounded.

AIDS stands in a symbolic (and thus also contemporaneous) relationship with the radioactive threat. With 'modern' humanity having turned away, at so much cost to itself, from the worlds of the invisible, the intangible, the numinous and the unconscious, those self-same worlds, so long supposed to be 'non-existent', are now striking back. In the process they are once again teaching humanity the primal terror which in antiquity it was the job of every demon, ghost, raging divinity and loathsome horror from the kingdom of the unseen to bring home to people at large.

The sex-drive, it is well known, has a great, even overwhelming power over human beings, with the capacity either to release or to bind according to the level on which it operates. It is certainly not for us to denigrate and repress sexuality all over again: the task which assuredly does face us, though, is that of bringing a sexuality that is seen in purely physical terms back into balance with that capacity for spiritual encounter which we call 'love' for short.

Let us sum up, then:

Sexuality and love are the two poles of a single theme whose name is 'the union of opposites'.

Sexuality is concerned with physicality; love with the other person's soul.

Sexuality and love need to be balanced out – that is, kept in equilibrium.

Psychological encounter (love) is apt to be experienced as dangerous and charged with fear because it throws the boundaries of our own ego into question. Any one-sided overemphasis on physical sexuality causes love to decline into the shadows. In such cases sexuality has a tendency to become aggressive and wounding (instead of the psychological boundaries of the *I*, it is the boundaries of the body that start to be penetrated – blood starts to flow).

AIDS is the final upshot of love that has fallen into the shadows. What AIDS does is to dissolve the boundaries of the *I* at the bodily level, so causing us to experience physically the fear of love that we have been avoiding at the psychological level.

Death, too, is ultimately the physical expression of love, in that it embodies our total sacrifice and surrender of the *I*'s separateness (compare the message of Christianity). But then death is only the start of a change, the beginning of a metamorphosis.

Sixteen

What to Do?

After all our many reflections designed to help patients learn how to understand the message of their symptoms a little, one is still left asking, 'How does knowing all this help me get better? What do I have to do now?' Our sole answer to such questions consists of just two words: 'Look within!' This exhortation will at first sight be regarded by most people as banal, simplistic and impractical. After all, surely we all want to do something about it, to change ourselves, to change anything and everything: what difference is looking within likely to make? In this constant desire to change things lies one of the greatest dangers along our way. For in reality there is absolutely nothing to change – apart from our way of seeing things. That is why our prescription simply boils down to 'Look within'.

There is nothing whatever that we can do in this universe other than learn to see – yet of all things this is the hardest. All development is based simply and solely on a change of viewpoint: everything else is merely a function of the new way of seeing. If, for example, we compare today's stage of technical development with that of the Middle Ages, the sole difference is that in the interim we have learnt to see new laws and potentialities in the world around us. Those laws and potentialities themselves were all there ten thousand years ago – but nobody was aware of them at the time. We always like to imagine that we are creating something new, and are consequently proud to talk about our 'inventions'. But this is to ignore the fact that all we can ever do is discover, not invent. All thoughts and ideas are potentially already there: it is just that we need time to assimilate them.

Harsh though it may sound to those who are anxious to improve the world, there is absolutely nothing in this world to improve or change, apart from our own way of seeing things. Thus it is that even the most complex problems always ultimately boil down to the old formula 'Know thyself!' So difficult and demanding is this in practice, though, that we constantly do our utmost to develop the most complex theories and systems for understanding and changing others, our relationships and the world around us. Following all this investment it is then pretty annoying to see all these over-inflated theories, systems and endeavours swept aside and replaced by the simple concept of self-knowledge. The concept, it is true, may seem simple – but translating it into practice certainly is not.

In this connection Jean Gebser writes in *Verfall und Teilhabe*:

> There is no way in which the much-needed changes to the world and to humanity will be achieved by trying to improve either. Those who do try to do so are merely using their struggle to improve the world as a way of avoiding improving themselves. They are playing the usual deplorable, if thoroughly human, game of demanding of others what one is too lazy to carry out oneself. Yet such illusory success as they achieve does not absolve them of having betrayed not only the world, but themselves too.

All that we need to do to improve ourselves, in fact, is to learn to see ourselves as we really are! But knowing ourselves does not mean knowing our ego. The 'I' is to the self as a glass of water is to the ocean. Our 'I' makes us sick: the self is whole. The way to healing is the way that leads out of the 'I' to the self, out of prison into freedom, out of polarity into unity. When a given symptom indicates to me what I (among others) still lack in order to be free, then it is for me to learn to see what is wrong, or lacking, and to accept it into my conscious *I*-dentification. The aim of our interpretations thus far has been to make us all look at what we otherwise normally *over*-look. Once we have seen it, all we have to do is not lose sight of it again – indeed, to look at it ever more closely. It is only constant, attentive observation that can overcome all the obstacles and encourage the growth of the love that is necessary if we are finally to assimilate what we have newly discovered. Merely to contemplate the shadow is to illumine it.

It is an entirely mistaken – if common – reaction to try to get rid of whatever issue is revealed by the symptom as quickly as possible. Thus, a person who has suddenly been horrified to discover his or her unconscious aggression may well ask, 'How can I get rid of this awful aggression again?' The answer is, 'You can't. Just enjoy it while it lasts!' It is precisely this desire to be rid of things that leads to a build-up of the shadow and makes us *un-whole*: seeing aggression for what it is, on the other hand, makes us *whole*. Those who regard this latter as dangerous are forgetting that an issue or principle does not disappear merely because we look the other way.

There is no such thing as a dangerous principle: all that is dangerous is a force that lacks any effective counterforce. Every principle is neutralised by its opposite. It is only in isolation that any principle is dangerous. Heat by itself is just as much a danger to life as unmitigated cold. In isolation, gentleness is no more noble than harshness. Only when the forces are in balance can tranquillity reign. The great difference between the 'way of the world' and the 'way of the wise' is that 'the world' always tries to bring just *one* pole into manifestation, whereas the 'wise' favour the mid-point between the two poles. Once we have grasped the fact that humanity is a microcosm, we gradually lose our fear of discovering *all* the various principles within ourselves.

If we discover in a symptom a principle that we are lacking, it is sufficient to learn to love that symptom, for it is a living manifestation of whatever is missing. If we are constantly itching with impatience to get rid of the symptom, we have simply not yet understood this concept. The symbol is a living manifestation of the shadow-principle in question – so, if we are to affirm this principle, we can hardly be fighting the symptom at the same time. Here, then, is one key to the answer. *Merely accepting the symptom renders it superfluous.* Resistance just results in counter-resistance. The symptom is only likely to disappear once it has become of no consequence to the patient. This lack of consequence is an indication that the patient has grasped the validity of the principle manifested by the symptom and has duly accepted it. The only way this can be achieved is by 'looking within'.

To avoid any misunderstanding at this point, it needs to be made clear once again that we are speaking here of illness at the content-level, and are not trying to lay down the law about what should be done on the practical level. Investigation of the content of symptoms does not necessarily forbid, prevent or render superfluous the adoption of any given functional measure. Our dealings with polarity should already have made clear our determination to replace every 'either/or' with a 'both/and'. Thus, in the case of a perforated stomach-ulcer, the question we would ask is not, 'Shall we interpret it, or shall we operate?' Far from making it superfluous, the one merely makes sense of the other for the first time. By itself an operation soon loses any sense it may have if the patient has failed to grasp its meaning

– while interpretation by itself is equally senseless if the patient has already died. At the same time the fact should not be overlooked that the vast majority of symptoms are not life-threatening, so that in such cases the question as to whether or not to adopt given functional measures is somewhat less urgent.

Functional measures, however, are never of any consequence to the subject of healing, irrespective of whether they work or not. Healing can only take place within our consciousness. It remains an open question, however, whether individual patients are capable in practice of ever becoming truly honest with themselves. Actual experience makes one sceptical. Even people who have engaged in a life-long struggle for self-awareness and self-knowledge often stay remarkably blind to certain of their own weak points. To this extent there are limitations to any individual's ability to apply the interpretations advanced in this book to his or her own particular case. Often it will be necessary to subject ourselves to more extensive and deep-reaching procedures if we are finally to encounter what we have hitherto done our best to avoid noticing. These ways of breaking through people's personal blind-spots are what are nowadays referred to as 'psychotherapy'.

Here we regard it as important to dispose straight away of the old preconception that psychotherapy is just a way of treating psychologically disturbed people or symptoms. This view may well have some validity in respect of strongly symptom-orientated methods (behavioural therapy, for instance), but it is certainly inapplicable to cases involving depth-psychology or transpersonally orientated approaches. Ever since the rise of psychoanalysis, psychotherapy has striven to promote self-knowledge and to make conscious the contents of the unconscious. From psychotherapy's point of view, there is nobody so healthy as not to be in urgent need of psychotherapy. The gestalt therapist Erving Polster once wrote, 'Therapy is too valuable to be reserved just for those who are ill.' It sounds somewhat harsher, perhaps, when we ourselves express the same view in the words: 'Illness is in our nature.'

Becoming conscious is the sole detectable purpose of our incarnation. Yet it is astonishing how little most people worry about this single most important issue in their lives. It is not without some irony that people devote so much care and attention to their bodies, notwithstanding the fact that these will all one day fall victim to the worms. The fact that all the rest, too, will one day have to be left behind (family, money, house, reputation, the lot) is a piece of news that likewise really ought to have got about by now. The only thing that survives the grave is consciousness itself – yet that is the last thing that anybody worries about. Consciousness is the goal of our very existence. It is this goal alone that serves the universe as a whole.

In all epochs people have sought to develop aids to help them on their painful path towards self-awareness and self-discovery. Here we may think of yoga, Zen, Sufism, Kabbala, magic and various other systems and disciplines. Their methods and practices are various, but their goal is the same – the perfection and liberation of humanity. The most recent offspring of this family, psychology and psychotherapy, grew out of the Western, scientifically orientated outlook of our own time. Blinded initially by its own youthful arrogance and hubris, psychology overlooked the fact that what it was only just starting to investigate was something that had long since been known about much more fully and in greater detail. Yet just as one cannot deny a child its own development, so psychology, too, had to experience things for itself until it gradually found its way into the mainstream of great doctrines concerning the human soul.

In this the real pioneers have been the psychotherapists, for everyday practical work corrects any theoretical imbalances a good deal more quickly than mere statistics and experimental hypotheses. As a result, we today are seeing in the application of psychotherapy a great confluence of ideas and methods drawn from all cultures, epochs and approaches. People everywhere are striving to forge a new synthesis of the many venerable forms of experience gained on the path to self-awareness. Nobody should be discouraged by the fact that any process as vehement as this is bound to produce a good deal of rubbish too.

For more and more contemporary people, psychotherapy is becoming a useful tool for experiencing their own psyche and so for getting to know themselves better. Psychotherapy produces no illuminati – but then neither does any other technique. The actual path leading to the goal is long and hard and only ever accessible to a few. Yet every step in the direction of greater consciousness is progress, and fulfils the requirements of development. Thus, while nobody should overdo their expectations of psychotherapy, it still represents one of today's best ways of becoming more conscious and more honest with ourselves.

When we, as authors of this book, speak of psychotherapy, we cannot help but take as our main starting-point the method that we ourselves have been using for some years, known as 'reincarnation therapy'. Since this concept was first made public in 1976 (Dethlefsen, T.: *Das Erlebnis der Wiedergeburt*), the term has frequently been taken over and used for all kinds of different therapeutic undertakings, so clouding the meaning of the term and leading to a whole variety of extraneous associations. Consequently we would regard it as appropriate at this point to offer a few explanatory words on the subject of reincarnation therapy, even though we do not intend to go into concrete detail about it.

Every preconception that a client has about a therapy actually gets in the way of it. Any *pre*-conception stands *in front of* the truth and hides it from view. Therapy is essentially a gamble, and needs to be experienced as such. The aim of therapy is to get people out of their anxious rigidity and their constant struggle for security and to involve them in the process of change. Moreover, therapy can have no firm manifesto of its own if it is not to run the risk of trampling on the patient's own individuality. For all these reasons we are not in the habit of supplying very much at all in the way of concrete information about reincarnation therapy. We do not talk about it: we simply do it. The only regrettable thing is that this vacuum is then liable to be filled with the suppositions, theories and opinions of people who actually have no idea of what our therapy involves.

It should already have become clear from the theoretical part of our book what, among other things, reincarnation therapy is *not*: in no way are we seeking the causes for any given symptom in previous lives. Reincarnation therapy is not just a version of psychoanalysis or primal scream therapy extended back in time. At the same time, though, it does not follow from this that there is absolutely no technique used in reincarnation therapy that is not also used in other therapies. On the contrary, reincarnation therapy is an extremely sophisticated concept which, on the practical level, has room for a good many well-tried techniques. But then technical variety is merely part of the natural armoury of any good therapist, and is no substitute for therapy itself. Psychotherapy is much more than applied technique – which is why psychotherapy is all but unteachable. The essential aspects of psychotherapy elude all description. It is a great mistake to assume that one can achieve the self-same results merely by aping the externals closely enough. Forms are vehicles for content – yet there are also such things as empty forms. Psychotherapy – just like any other esoteric technique, of course – soon turns into a farce once the forms lose their content.

Reincarnation therapy owes its name to the fact that becoming aware of past incarnations and living them through is something that figures large in our form of therapy. Since working on one's incarnations is for many people something pretty exotic in itself, there are a good many who fail to realise that becoming aware of one's incarnations belongs purely to the technical and formal side of our therapy, and is far from being an end in itself. By itself, living out one's incarnations is not a therapy, any more than is mere screaming; but both can be used therapeutically. The reason why we make people aware of their incarnations is not that we regard it as important or exciting to know who or what any given person was previously: we use incarnations simply because we can currently think of no better tool for attaining the goal of our therapy.

We have shown exhaustively in this book how people's problems always lie in their shadow. For this reason the encounter with the shadow and its gradual assimilation is the central plank in reincarnation therapy. Indeed our technique makes it possible to encounter the great karmic shadow which to a degree puts even this life's biographical shadow in the shade. Getting to grips with the shadow is certainly not easy – yet it is the only way that leads to healing in the true sense of the word. However, it would be pointless to say any more here about the encounter with the shadow and its assimilation, since the experiencing of deep, spiritual realities cannot be reproduced in words. What people's incarnations offer in this connection is a chance to experience and integrate the shadow while fully identifying themselves with it, in a way that other techniques are hard put to emulate.

We do not work with memories: instead, the various incarnations actually become present experience. This is possible because time does not exist outside our own consciousness. Time is merely *one* possible way of looking at what happens. We know from physics that time can be transformed into space – for space is the *other* way of looking at the relationships between things. If we apply this transformation to the problem of successive incarnations, the usual *one-thing-after-another-ness* turns into a *one-thing-alongside-another-ness* – or, to put it another way, the temporal chain of lives turns into a simultaneous, spatially parallel experience. Granted, the spatial interpretation of human incarnations is neither more right nor wrong than the temporal model – both ways of looking at things are perfectly legitimate subjective points of view for human consciousness to take up (compare the wave-versus-particle argument in the case of light). Every attempt actually to experience that which is spatially synchronous, however, immediately turns space back into time. To take an example: in a given space there are many different radio programmes going on at any one time. If, however, we want to listen to these simultaneously-present radio programmes, it immediately becomes a case of *one-thing-after-another*. This involves tuning the receiver to various frequencies in turn, whereupon the apparatus will put us in contact with various programmes in accordance with the particular resonance-frequencies selected. If we now replace the radio-receiver in our example with human consciousness itself, the respective resonance-frequencies instead come up with corresponding incarnations.

In reincarnation therapy we get our clients to turn a deaf ear to their present frequency (their current identification), so letting go of it and leaving space for other resonances to appear. The moment they do so, other incarnations come through – incarnations that are experienced as being just as 'real' as the life with which the client has identified to date. Since the 'other lives' or identifications exist simultaneously and in parallel, they are equally capable of being experienced with all the perceptions. The 'third programme' is no more remote than the 'first' or 'second' programmes: true, we can only perceive one of them at a time, but we can switch between them at will. By analogy with the radio, then, we go on to switch the consciousness-frequency around and so change the particular 'angle of incidence' and resonance-frequency.

In reincarnation therapy we deliberately play with time. We 'pump' time, as it were, into the various structures of consciousness, so causing them to swell up and become visible; and we stop time so as to make it possible to experience the fact that everything constantly belongs in the here and now. Often one hears the criticism that reincarnation therapy consists of a pointless rummaging around in earlier lives, when people's problems really need to be solved in the here and now. In reality, however, what we do is gradually to dissolve the illusion of time and causality and confront clients with the *eternal* here and now. We know of no other therapy that so mercilessly removes all the projection-screens and hands responsibility for everything back to the individual concerned.

What reincarnation therapy attempts to set in train is a psychological process, with the important thing being the process, and not the intellectual classification or interpretation of what is going on. That is why we have devoted the concluding section of this book to a discussion of psychotherapy, for there is a widely held view that psychotherapy is just for healing psychological disorders and symptoms. Even today, people confronted with purely physical symptoms seldom get around to thinking of the possibility of psychotherapy. In the light both of our general outlook and of our experience, however, psychotherapy is the one and only approach that actually offers any real promise of physical healing.

As we approach the end of this particular book, it should no longer be necessary for us to explain the grounds for this view. Anybody who has developed an eye for the way in which every physical process and symptom is an expression of a psychological event will know by now that, by the same token, it is only processes at the level of consciousness that can resolve whatever problems come to light in bodily form. Consequently we know of no indications or contra-indications for psychotherapy. All we know is people who are ill, and who are being impelled towards healing by their symptoms. It is the job of psychotherapy to help people undertake this process of development and change. That is why in psychotherapy we ally ourselves with our clients' symptoms and help the latter attain their goal – for the body is always right. Academic medicine does the opposite – it allies itself with patients *against* their symptoms. We always stand on the side of the shadow and help it to emerge into the light. We wage no war against illness and its symptoms, but instead endeavour to use it as a point of leverage for healing.

Illness is both humanity's great opportunity and its most precious commodity. Illness is our personal teacher and guide on the road to wholeness. Various paths to this goal are available to us, most of them difficult and complicated, yet the most obvious and personal of these for the most part goes unheeded and ignored – namely illness. This is the path that is least susceptible to the mirages of self-delusion. That, no doubt, is why it is also so unpopular. In therapy, as in this book, it is our aim to rescue illness from its usual, narrow connotations and to reveal its true relationship to our experience as human beings. Those who decline to go along with us as we take the decisive step into this alternative frame of reference will inevitably misunderstand everything we have said. Those, on the other hand, who have managed to grasp illness's role as a path in its own right will open up for themselves a whole world of new insights. Our way of dealing with illness makes life neither easier nor healthier; rather it is our aim to give people the courage to look our polar world's conflicts and problems honestly in the eye. It is our purpose to unmask the delusion of a world that is not only hostile to any kind of conflict, but then goes on to imagine that an earthly paradise can somehow be constructed on the basis of sheer dishonesty.

Hermann Hesse once said, 'Problems are not there in order to be solved: they are merely the poles between which life's necessary tensions can arise.' The solution lies beyond polarity – yet in order to get there it is necessary to unite the poles and reconcile the opposites. This difficult art of uniting the opposites can be mastered only by those who have fully acquainted themselves with both poles. One then has to have the courage to experience and integrate those poles. *Solve et coagula*, as the ancient texts have it – release and bind. We have to start by differentiating, by experiencing disunity and division, before we can venture onwards to the Great Work of the Alchemical Wedding that is the union of the opposites. So it is that we have first to descend deep into the polarity of the world of matter, into physicality, illness, sin and guilt, in order to discover in the darkest night of the soul, in the deepest despair and *dis-traction*, that light of *real-isation* which enables us to see our path through suffering and torture for what it is – a game pregnant with meaning that can help us find our way back to where in reality we always were: in the Oneness itself.

> I have known good and evil,
> sin and virtue, right and wrong;
> I have judged and been judged;
> I have passed through birth and death,
> joy and sorrow, heaven and hell;
> and in the end I realised
> that I am in everything
> and everything is in me.

Hazrat Inayat Khan
(retranslated from the German)

A List of Psychological Equivalents of Organs and Parts of the Body in Common Idioms

back	uprightness
bladder	release of pressure
blood	life-force, vitality
bones	firmness, fulfilment of norms
ears	obedience
eyes	insight
feet	understanding, steadfastness, rootedness, humility, submissiveness
finger- and toenails	aggression
gall-bladder	aggression
genitals	sexuality
gums	native confidence
hair	freedom, power
hands	comprehension, ability to act
heart	ability to love, emotion
kidneys	partnership
knees	humility, submissiveness
large intestine	greed, the unconscious
limbs	mobility, flexibility, activity
liver	discrimination, philosophy, religion
lungs	contact, communication, freedom
mouth	readiness to accept
muscles	mobility, flexibility, activity
neck	fear, anxiety
nose	power, pride, sexuality
penis	power
skin	delimitation, norms, contact, tenderness
small intestine	processing, analysis
stomach	feelings, receptivity
teeth	aggression, vitality
throat	fear, anxiety
vagina	self-surrender

Index of Symptoms

The index which follows is designed to help readers look up given symptoms quickly in the text. In those cases where a symptom is discussed directly in the text, the corresponding page number is shown in the normal way. At the same time there are further symptoms to which an interpretation applies which is the same as, or similar to, that given for the symptoms actually discussed: these, too, are therefore included in the index. In such cases reference is made to those symptoms that are analogous to those in question ('see...'): where more than one page number is given, this represents an invitation to the reader to put together his or her own interpretation by reading up several different aspects of the case (for example, 'inflammation' plus the particular organ involved). The index includes both common and technical terms.